Manual of Cancer Pain

W0227779

Edited by:

F. DE CONNO, MD
and
A. CARACENI, MD
Istituo Nazionale per lo Studio e la Cura dei Tumori, Milan, Italy

Editorial Board:

CARL JOHAN FURST, MD
Stockholms Sjukhem, Stockholm, Sweden

JOHAN MENTEN, MD
University Hospital, Leuven, Belgium

PHILIPPE POULAIN, MD
Institut Gustave Roussy, Villejuif-Cedex, France

JORDI ROCA I CASAS, MD
Hospital de la Santa Creu, Barcelona, Spain

PAT WEBB
Trinity Hospice, London, Great Britain

KLUWER ACADEMIC PUBLISHERS
DORDRECHT / BOSTON / LONDON

Library of Congress Cataloging-in-Publication Data

A C.I.P. Catalogue record for this book is avaliable from the Library of Congress.

ISBN-13: 978-0-7923-4202-1   e-ISBN-13: 978-94-009-1762-0
DOI: 10.1007978-94-009-1762-0

Published by Kluwer Academic Publishers BV,
PO Box 17, 3300 AA Dordrecht, The Netherlands.

Kluwer Academic Publishers BV incorporates
the publishing programmes of
D. Reidel, Martinus Nijhoff, Dr W. Junk and MTP Press.

Sold and distributed in the United States and Canada
by Kluwer Academic Publishers, PO Box 358,
Accord Station, Hingham, MA 02018-0358, USA

In all other countries, sold and distributed
by Kluwer Academic Publishers Group, Distribution Center,
PO Box 322, 3300 AH Dordrecht, The Netherlands

Printed on acid-free paper

Foreword

Pain in oncology, and especially in patients with advanced disease, is an essential issue which cannot be overlooked.

Today, pain is worldwide recognised as a very complex symptom which includes different aspects such as somatic, spiritual, social and psychological pain.

Practical and scientific knowledge of pain in cancer should be part of the pre- and post-training of general practitioners, oncologists and nurses.

This manual reflects the opinion of different authors and contributors to pain clinic. These guidelines cover different aspects of cancer pain. It responds to a need for information, education and training in the field of diagnosis and treatment of cancer pain. The reader will find useful information and suggestions as how to diagnose and treat pain from a pharmacological and surgical point of view.

Pain treatment is a very important part of quality of life: due to its relevance, we think that this manual will be a very useful tool for all health professionals, and we are grateful to Drs De Conno and Caraceni for their generous contribution in making this effort successful.

Alberto Costa
Director
European School of Oncology

Acknowledgements

The authors and the European School of Oncology would like to express their thanks to Janssen Pharmaceutica who have made the printing of this booklet possible.

Preface

Cancer pain is still undertreated but instruments exist for controlling this feared symptom of advanced cancer. It is therefore the responsibility of medicine to apply the existing instruments.

This manual covers basic information which should enable the successful diagnosis and treatment of 90% of patients with pain due to cancer. Our aim has been, not to trivialize the problem which remains complex and in some cases difficult to solve, but to help all health care professionals involved in the care of cancer patients who are not pain specialists in understanding and managing most of the situations they will see in their clinical practice. Other relevant subjects should also be considered such as the psychosocial dimension of suffering and pain in children with cancer, which deserve to be reviewed separately and could well be the subject of other similar manuals.

For this reason we have summarized detailed diagnostic and therapeutic aspects together with simple guidelines to give the reader an idea of the different levels of complexity entailed by the comprehensive management of cancer pain.

F. De Conno and A. Caraceni

Contents

1. INTRODUCTION

Pain is a major symptom in cancer. It has been estimated that about 30% of patients undergoing active treatment and 70% of patients with advanced untreatable disease suffer pain due to tumor progression (1-3). The availability of guidelines (4, 5) and accumulating clinical experience has greatly improved the possibility of satisfactory pain control for most patients with advanced cancer (6). It is less clear how guidelines and educational resources impacted on daily practice in the oncology clinics and wards and at the community level. Recent surveys found that cancer pain is less than optimally controlled (7, 8) and that physicians' knowledge and attitudes in pain management are likely to contribute to under-treatment (9, 10). Other contributing factors should be also considered including patient-related barriers (11) and pain pathophysiology. Difficult pain problems associated with rapidly progressive disease, very severe pain, or pain syndromes relatively resistant to opioid analgesics can be an obstacle to good pain relief in a proportion of patients which is yet unknown, and estimated to range from 20% to 30% according to different surveys (6, 12).

The aim of a practical manual should be to give a synthesis of standard approaches to aggressive and comprehensive pain assessment and management using the available resources for common pain problems and to highlight potential alternatives in recognizing difficult pain syndromes requiring more specialized multidisciplinary evaluation.

2. PAIN ASSESSMENT

2.1. Emergency pain

Assessment of pain is of paramount importance in implementing effective treatment. The severity of pain will guide immediate or delayed intervention. It is common to see patients referred for pain control who are in excruciating pain at the time of referral. These situations are to be seen as emergencies and should be treated accordingly before beginning the process of routine assessment and evaluation. A rational approach to emergency cancer related pain includes a brief assessment of the situation using all available information from the patient, the chart and the referring physician, in order to exclude the most important complications. We designed an algorithm (Fig. 1 and Table 1) to highlight the main characteristics of these difficult situations with the aim of underlining that pain needs to be under control before proceeding to order diagnostic tests or to suggest a new analgesic regimen or palliative therapy such as radiation. Pain control will allow patients to undergo imaging and treatments which would be otherwise impossible. This approach requires specialized personnel available in the radiology or radiotherapy suites to administer and titrate analgesics and evaluate effects. Only preemptive assessment can allow timely intervention and pain control.

2.2. Clinical assessment

Pain in cancer always needs to be characterized accurately. Clinical evaluation will disclose the cause and the pathophysiology of pain in most cases. The patient's complaint should, as a rule, be believed. Patients are usually very accurate and precise in describing their pain and its characteristics. Therefore first, listen to the patient and take a complete history of the pain in the context of the history of the oncological disease. Since more than one pain with different pathophysiologies is common, each pain needs to be assessed looking at site, aggravating and relieving factors, radiation and temporal factors (acute, subacute, chronic, intermittent, exacerbation, breakthrough pains). In fact 70% of patients with cancer pain present at least two pain sites (13) and about 60% experience episodes of breakthrough pain (14). A careful list of all previous treatments and their analgesic efficacy and side effects is very useful. Doses and modality of administration are to be reviewed since most often inadequate titration or less than optimal management of side effects is the cause for the premature conclusion that a given drug "does not work". Psychological and psychosocial history is part of the evaluation and is necessary to implement a comprehensive plan of care. A istory of alcohol and drug abuse should be sought. Physical examination should always include a neurological exam to evaluate the presence of neuropathic pain and of neurological complications of the disease. In a recent survey on 2266 cancer patients with pain 34% had a neuropathic pain (13). In another survey pain diagnosis led to the discovery of new lesions in 64% of cases and led to a specific palliative oncologic

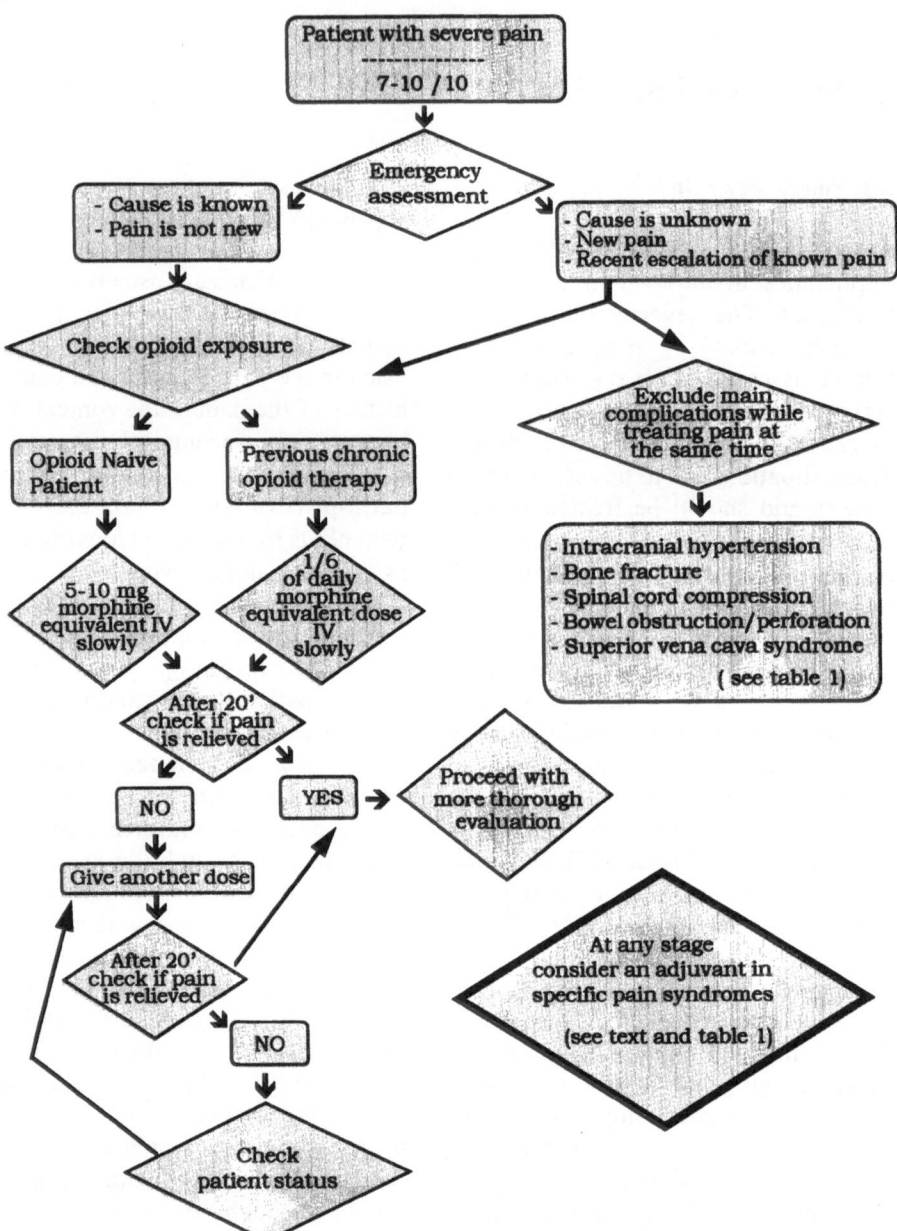

Figure 1. Algorithm for emergency pain treatment. Dose titration should start with 5 mg morphine equivalents in opioid naive patients ≥65 years of age and 10 mg in younger patients. Clinical judgement should guide the use of lower doses in frail, advanced patients no matter what their age.

Subsequent doses can be given monitoring patient status, i.e. sedation, respiratory rate and blood pressure. The use of an adjuvant can be suggested at different stages of the process if pain is relatively unresponsive to one or two opioid doses and requires expert advice.

Table 1. Pharmacological management of complications and specific pain conditions*

Bone fracture	NSAID IV (e.g. ketorolac 30 mg, naproxen 500 mg), evaluate operability
Spinal cord compression	Dexamethasone 10–100 mg IV (methylprednisolone 150 mg IV) (expert advice needed), emergency RT, evaluate operability
Bowel obstruction	Evaluate operability, pain can be managed with opioids
Superior vena cava syndrome	Dexamethasone 10 mg IV (methylprednisolone 150 mg IV)
Intracranial hypertension	Dexamethasone 10 mg IV (methylprednisolone 150 mg IV) (if impending cerebral herniation 100 mg can be given), mannitol 20%
	Opioids are not indicated
Refractory neuropathic pain (e.g. herpes zoster, lancinating nerve pain)	Dexamethasone 10 mg IV (methylprednisolone 150 mg IV)
	Phenytoin 1000 mg IV load (expert advice needed)
	Lidocaine 5 mg/kg IV infusion (expert advice needed)
Pain sustained by inflammatory process (e.g. bone metastases, pleurisy)	NSAID IV (e.g. ketorolac 30 mg IV, naproxen 500 mg)

* Treatments to be considered in all cases of proven complications and as potential adjuvants for very difficult pain conditions with the characteristics listed above

treatment (radiotherapy) in about 20%. More than 50% of all the new diagnoses were neurologic pain syndromes (15). New imaging tests can be ordered following careful assessment and results have to be personally reviewed to obtain all useful information about pain etiology.

2.3. Pain measurement

Pain severity can be assessed by several methods. It is however important that pain intensity is measured and recorded to help in monitoring therapy results and to improve communication with the patient. Most patients will learn to use simple pain scales even when they may look unfamiliar from the beginning. Clinician–patient communication on pain can be simplified and improved by the introduction of these simple scales (16). Other patients can find it difficult for cultural and individual reasons to use any kind of scale and this has also to be considered.

Different pain measurement tools have been validated for use in cancer patients with pain. They can be divided in two main categories: intensity scales and multidimensional questionnaires.

Intensity scales are visual analogue scales (VAS), numerical scales (NRS) (usually from 0 to 10) and verbal rating scales (VRS). These methods behave very similarly in the clinical situation (17). VAS can be difficult to use with less educated patients and with the elderly, 0 to 10 NRS seem to have common meaning across cultures while keeping some desirable psychometric properties if compared with VRS.

Pain is a multidimensional experience. Two or three dimension models have been proposed: pain intensity and aversiveness or unpleasantness are used to explain the variability of the pain experience according to one model (18). Another model explains pain variability as due to the existence of a sensory discriminative dimension, an affective-emotional and a cognitive component (19). In clinical practice we have to consider that pain intensity alone may not be sufficient to evaluate treatment efficacy and that we need to know how much a given pain level bothers the patient, which is the level of pain that can be considered tolerable, what corresponds to satisfactory pain relief, how pain interferes with quality of life and where would the patient place himself along the trade off between pain relief and side effects.

Several instruments are available for the multidimensional evaluation of cancer pain, the best known of which are the McGill Pain Questionnaire (20), the Brief Pain Inventory (21), and the Memorial Pain Assessment Card (22). All of them are valid and reliable. The Memorial Pain Assessment Card proved particularly useful in controlled clinical trials on the clinical pharmacology of opioids.

The McGill Pain Questionnaire is a complex tool, based on the use of differ-ent pain descriptors which should reflect the evaluation of different pain dimensions with an intensity ranking within each dimension. It has been translated in several national versions, but their equivalency with the English version has not been well demonstrated. In our own experience it was not possible to demonstrate the superiority of this tool, in its Italian version, over more simple scales (VAS, NRS, VRS) in evaluating pain control after implementing treatment (23). At the moment it should be considered an important research tool (24) while waiting for more experience for its use in the clinical management of cancer pain.

The Brief Pain Inventory (BPI) is based on 0 to 10 scales evaluating pain intensity and interference with function (7 areas of psychosocial and physical activities). It has also been translated and validated in several languages (Chinese, French, Italian, Philippino and Spanish) and proved to be valid and reliable across translations (18, 25). The use of the BPI in large multicenter trials allowed identification of pain levels which represent clinically important cut-offs because of their interference with function. When pain intensity reaches a level of 5 it starts to interfere significantly with life activities and when it reaches a level of 7 its interference with function again rises significantly (18).

These results can improve our use of intensity scales in allowing an operational definition of "significant" pain when pain intensity scores $\geqslant 5$ over 10.

Pain relief scales are also often used (from 0 to 100%) but they are only partially associated with pain intensity measures and seem indeed more associated with measures of mood and psychological distress (22, 23, 26). For this reason it is not totally clear at the moment which is the best way to use pain relief scales in clinical practice and what they are actually measuring.

The following steps need however to be considered when choosing one method for systematic patient assessment:

1. Establish frequency of evaluation and method.

2. Establish time referral: average measures of last 24 h pain or last week pain have been used but the clinical context should dictate the most appropriate method, "pain now" is certainly the most reliable of all measures.

3. Pain quality and intensity in cancer change in time and breakthrough pain is very common. Episodes of breakthrough pain should be evaluated aside to baseline pain. Only one scoring method (27) attempted to integrate in one measure different

pain intensities with their respective duration over 24 h to calculate a single score without however being able to show a clear clinical benefit from the method compared with simpler scales (23).

4. Different pain sites are common in cancer with different pathophysiologies, severity and responses to treatment and a body chart showing pain sites should also be part of the regular assessment. Worst pain intensity is probably the most important clinical variable.

5. Pain intensity measures should however be visible in patients' charts and be part of routine patient evaluation in oncology (16, 28). Standard requirements for improving quality of patients' care have been published which require the adoption of a pain measurement scale and its visibility in the chart among the essential (29) changes to be implemented for better pain control.

3. PATHOPHYSIOLOGY OF PAIN IN CANCER

Pain in patients with cancer is due to the tumor in about 70% of cases, to anti-neoplastic treatments in more than 20% of cases, and is not related to the tumor nor to treatments in less than 10% of cases (30). Acute, subacute and chronic pain syndromes can be due to surgery, radio- and chemotherapy (Tables 2 and 3). The differential diagnosis between tumor recurrence and post-treatment

Table 2. Acute and subacute pain syndromes in cancer patients associated with various treatments

Intercostal pleural catheter

Chemical pleurodesis

Pleural alcoholization

Biliary catheterization, biliary stents

Percutaneous nephrostomy

Esophageal dilatation with endoprosthesis

Special chemotherapy modalities
- Tumor chemoembolization (especially of hepatic lesions)
- Hepatic artery perfusion
- Intraperitoneal chemotherapy
- Hyperthermic limb perfusion chemotherapy
- Mesenteric perfusion chemotherapy
- Intrathecal methotrexate-induced meningismus

Systemic chemotherapy
- Mucositis
- Steroid pseudorheumatism
- Jaw, abdominal and limb pains following neurotoxic agents (vincristine, vinblastine, vindesine, vinorelbine, paclitaxel)
- Diffuse bone pain associated with transretinoic acid or with GCSF administration
- Transretinoic acid headache

Hormonal therapy
- LHRH associated flare of pain in prostate cancer
- Hormone induced pain flare in breast cancer

Bone marrow transplant
- Graft versus host disease

Radiation therapy
- Oropharyngeal mucositis
- Esophagitis
- Acute radiation enteritis-proctitis
- Early onset brachial plexopathy
- Cystitis induced by chemo or radiotherapy

Table 3. Chronic pain syndromes related to cancer treatments

Post-surgical pain syndrome related to non-healing incision

Post-surgical neuropathic syndromes
- Post-mastectomy
- Post-axillary dissection
- Post-inguinal dissection
- Post-thoracotomy
- Postradical neck dissection
- Postnephrectomy
- Post-limb amputation
- Post-rectal amputation
- Stump pain

Post-radiotherapy syndromes
- Radiation enteritis and cystitis
- Radiation dermatitis and muscle fibrosis
- Osteoradionecrosis
- Radiation fibrosis of brachial or lumbosacral plexus
- Radiation myelopathy
- Radiation-induced peripheral nerve tumors

Post-chemotherapy syndromes
- Aseptic necrosis of bone
- Diffuse polyneuropathy
- Steroid pseudorheumatism

syndrome is an important aspect of pain evaluation but in most cases it is relatively simple. The cases requiring a more careful assessment are described below.

The pathophysiology of cancer pain is extremely variable. The tumor can involve visceral, somatic and nervous structures either at the same time or at different times. This can be due to progressive tumor invasion or compression from the tissue where the tumor originally developed. The same pattern can be seen for metastases.

The International Association for the Study of Pain defines pain as "an unpleasant sensory and emotional experience associated with actual or potential tissue damage, or described in terms of such damage". Most commonly pain is perceived when that part of the peripheral nervous system which is called nociceptive is activated. Nociception is the activity in the nervous system produced by tissue-damaging stimuli. Pain is the perception of nociception, and it is the product of the central nervous system integration of the nociceptive activity. Its relationship with the extent of tissue damage is usually evident in cancer but other factors may also be important. The complexity of the system in fact incorporates different levels of plasticity which are responsible for changes within the peripheral and the central nervous system due to chronic activation of nociceptors, to lesions of the nervous system itself or to psychological factors. These changes are grouped under the definition of non-nociceptive factors and are called neuropathic and psychological factors (31).

3.1. Nociceptive pain

Nociceptive pain is defined as pain that is believed to result from the activation of nociceptors in somatic or visceral structures. It is directly related to the location and extent of tissue damage. Nociceptive somatic pain is often described as sharp, aching, throbbing or pressure-like, while visceral pain is poorly localized and may be gnawing or cramping when due to involvement of a hollow viscus or aching or sharp when due to a lesion of an organ capsule or mesentery. Somatic nociceptive pain usually responds well to all forms of analgesic therapy, including non-opioid and opioid analgesics and anesthetic or neurosurgical approaches.

3.2. Neuropathic pain

Neuropathic pain results from changes in the physiological response of neurons in the central or peripheral somatosensory system due to chronic stimulation or to a lesion of the nervous tissue. The diagnosis is usually based on the findings of a neurological lesion and sensory abnormalities such as dysesthesia, allodynia or hyperalgesia (Table 4). The subjective perception often includes burning or stabbing sensations. Peripheral nerve lesions caused by tumor, surgery or chemotherapy are the most common substrate for neuropathic pain in cancer patients.

Neuropathic pain has a variable response to opioid analgesia (32). Recent data confirm that neuropathic pain does

Table 4. Common sensory neurological findings in neuropathic pain

Spontaneous pain
Burning, shooting, lancinating

Negative findings
Hypoesthesia to touch and vibratory stimulation
Hypoalgesia to pin prick
Hypoesthesia to thermal warm and cold stimuli
Enhanced thermal pain threshold to quantitative sensory testing

Positive findings
Paresthesias – abnormal non-painful sensations
Dysesthesias – abnormal uncomfortable sensations
Allodynia – painful sensation evoked by a non-noxious stimulus
Hyperalgesia – exaggerated response to a noxious stimulus
Hyperpthia – exaggerated painful response to a noxious or non-noxious stimulus (*Example*: when the burning pain evoked by light touching (= allodynia) outlasts for seconds or minutes the duration of the stimulus)

respond to opioid analgesia (33) and the diagnosis of neuropathic pain should not limit a therapeutic opioid trial in cancer patients. When looking at the overall population, patients with neuropathic cancer pain have a reduced opioid responsiveness in comparison to the pain syndromes related predominantly to nociceptive mechanisms, shifting to the right the dose response curve for opioids in these syndromes (34, 35). The classification of cancer pain as neuropathic is frequently unclearly defined (36). Clinical experience also suggests that neurolytic blockade of pain pathways may have limited value or is harmful in cases of neuropathic pain due to central mechanisms (37). Adjuvant analgesics (see below) play an important role in treating neuropathic pain.

3.3 Idiopathic pain

The definition of idiopathic pain is used to define pain of unknown origin. An example is psychogenic pain which is uncommon in cancer patients. It is very difficult to attribute pain to psychological factors in cancer unless detailed psychiatric evaluation yields a specific diagnosis. However a psychiatric diagnosis for the pain should be applied with extreme caution in patients with cancer. Cancer pain usually relates closely to the underlying organic pathology. Pain may occur before other clinical, biochemical or imaging data prove evidence of tumor growth and we commonly see an excessive use of the psychogenic issue in these cases.

Do not use placebo for assessing the nature of the pain.

The mechanism of placebo response is complex and is always active in any therapeutic setting, pharmacological and non-pharmacological, whether or not pain is the issue. There is no rational basis to using a placebo for clarifying the potential psychogenic nature of the patient's pain. Placebos should only be used only within controlled pharmacological trials.

4. CANCER PAIN SYNDROMES

On the basis of the most frequent clinical and instrumental findings a long list of pain syndromes have been described. A detailed description of these syndromes can be found elsewhere (38, 39).

It is very important to establish a diagnosis and to anticipate complications which will potentially need immediate reassessment. Pain is often the first symptom of these complications, as seen in Figure 1.

4.1. Bone pain

The most common cause of pain in cancer is bone invasion. Bone metastases occur in 30 to 70% of all patients with cancer.

The exact mechanism by which tumor growth in bone produces pain is unknown and probably involves stimulation of periosteal nociceptors via different mechanisms (40). Pain that is aggravated by weight bearing, movement and exercise is the result of an imbalance in the structural properties of the bone leading to activation of periosteal nociceptors. Pain on activity should always be regarded as a sign of abnormality of the osseous structures with a potential for fracture. Increasing pain in a weight bearing bone even in the absence of radiological signs of local progression should be viewed as a warning for potential imminent fracture.

Bone pain is often reported in the body area corresponding to the site of the underlying lesion. It can also be referred to distant cutaneous areas, e.g. hip pain referred to the knee (see below for the referral pattern of vertebral

pain), but it is always reproduced by direct stimulation over the involved bone.

A variety of bone pain syndromes can be found according to different tumors and their evolution (Table 5).

Table 5. Bone pain

Base of skull syndromes

Vertebral syndromes (including sacrum)

Diffuse bone pain
- Due to multiple bone metastases
- Due to bone marrow infiltration/ expansion

Focal bone pain
- Long bones
- Chest wall rib pain
- Infiltration of a joint (sacroiliac joint)
- Pelvic bony lesions

4.1.1. Bone marrow expansion and bone marrow infiltration syndrome

This kind of pain can be difficult to diagnose because X-ray and even MRI imaging are often difficult to interpretate. Pain can be generalized and migrating and often fluctuates in intensity with therapeutic interventions (chemotherapy and steroids). It is found with hematologic malignancies (especially acute leukemias) and rarely with diffuse marrow infiltration by solid tumors (breast, melanoma). The pain can be reported in the long bones but can also affect the spine. Local bone tenderness and referred pain are frequent findings.

4.1.2. Vertebral pain syndromes

The vertebrae are the most common sites of bone metastases; they are usually multiple and involve the vertebral body first. The thoracic spine is affected in more than two thirds of cases, the lumbosacral spine in 20% and the cervical spine in 10% of cases. Some tumors can invade the vertebrae from contiguous paraspinal sites as in sarcomas, paraspinal nodes or apical lung tumors.

Pain due to vertebral metastases with or without epidural spinal cord compression is worse in prone position than if seated; the opposite is true for herniated disc pain or facet joint disease. In the affected area the underlying spine is often tender and muscle spasm is observed. Often pain can be referred to the limbs from vertebral lesions and can be worsened by Lasegue's maneuver (straight leg raising test) without clinical evidence of a radiculopathy. Table 6 reports characteristic referrals of pain due to vertebral lesions at different levels.

The main complications of vertebral metastases are: vertebral collapse, radiculopathy and epidural spinal cord compression (ESCC).

Collapse of vertebral bodies is particularly frequent in the thoracic and lower lumbar (L5) spine. It can acutely aggravate the pain syndrome, impinge on the nerve roots, and cause skeletal deformities, implying a higher risk for ESCC or cauda equina compression.

Radiculopathies can develop at any level: the pain is felt on the spine, deep in the muscles innervated by the affected root and in the corresponding dermatome. The diagnosis of radiculopathy requires the association of sensory, motor and reflex findings. Pain pattern and pain provoking maneuvers can be very helpful in characterizing the pain pathophysiology. Pain is usually exacerbated by increasing intraspinal pressure by coughing, sneezing and straining. Direct straight leg raising tests (SLRT) may not be specific but a positive crossed SLRT is always a sign of radiculopathy.

4.1.3. Epidural spinal cord compression (ESCC)

ESCC is the most dangerous complication of vertebral metastases. It represents a catastrophe for the patient's quality of life. ESCC occurs in 5 to 10% of patients with cancer. In patients with solid tumors it is usually caused by the posterior extension of tumor into a vertebral body, but with other malignancies such as lymphoma, paragangliomas and neuroblastomas, invasion of the epidural space through the intervertebral foramina in the absence of a bone lesion is the predominant mechanism. If untreated, ESCC leads to paraplegia or quadriplegia. The rate of paralysis is related to the neurological status at the time of therapy and the histology of the primary tumor (41). Therefore early diagnosis of the etiology of the neck or back pain and prompt treatment are critical.

Pain characteristics coupled with the findings of clinical examination and plain radiographs can be used to judge the relative risk of epidural extension and therefore of cord compression (42). The clinical context will dictate the aggressiveness with which to pursue a definitive imaging of the spinal canal.

Table 6. Vertebral pain – pattern of referral

Vertebrae	Pain characteristics	Notes
C1-C2	Neck pain radiating to the vertex	Cord compression at cervico-medullary junction, life threatening complication
C3-C4	Neck pain, radiating to shoulders	
C5-C6	Neck, shoulder arm pain	Often associated with radiculopathy. If symptoms of radiculopathy are bilateral cord compression is very likely
C7-T2	Infrascapular pain, arm pain	Same as C5-C6 Often difficult to image on plain X-rays because of overlapping shoulder tissue
T3-T11	Middle dorsal pain can radiate to the chest	When bilateral, tight band like sensation, compression fracture very likely with epidural extension
T12-L1	Groin pain radiating to the genitals	In case of radiculopathy can be elicited by neck flexion
L2	Low back pain (LBP) Upper thigh	
L3	LBP Upper and external area of the thigh, knee	
L4-L5	LBP Pain below knee	Sudden increase of pain with impossibility of moving indicates vertebral body compression fracture
S1-S2	Sacral pain Posterior thigh, popliteal fossa	
S3-S5	Sacral pain Gluteal and perineal	Cauda equina compression main complication

4.1.1.1. Pain characteristics

Funicular characteristics of the pain, and Lhermitte's sign, are to be regarded as evidence of myelopathy and always require emergency imaging, as well as all cases with myelopathic symptoms. Funicular pain is a rare finding and results from damage to the ascending spinal tracts. It is felt as a cold unpleasant sensation in the extremities, or as poorly localized non-dermatomal dysesthesia located at some distance below the compression (43).

Lhermitte's sign consists of an electric shock-like sensation radiating down from the spine into the legs when bending the neck and is typical for cervical spinal cord demyelinating lesions of multiple sclerosis. It is not rare as an early symptom of ESCC due to cancer, where it has also been described with thoracic lesions as the first symptom of myelopathy (44).

Increasing local or radicular pain worsened by recumbency, sneezing, coughing or straining also bears a greater likelihood of ESSC (pain in "crescendo pattern"). A clinically defined radiculopathy is associated with epidural extension of tumor in 60% of cases (45, 46).

4.1.1.2. Radiographic characteristics

A radiographic abnormality can predict epidural invasion in 60% of the cases in patients with back pain and a normal neurologic exam. The association of clinical signs of radiculopathy and a radiographic lesion bring this percentage to 90% (45–47).

Epidural tumor was found in 87% of the cases where there was greater than 50% collapse of the vertebral body demonstrated on the plain radiographs, and in 31% of the cases with pedicle erosion (48).

In a study comparing bone scan results, only 17% of the cases with back pain, with a positive bone scan and a normal radiograph had epidural disease (47).

Lymphomas and pediatric tumors often infiltrate the epidural space via the neural foramina. In these populations radiographs can be normal in as many as 70% of patients (49, 50).

4.1.1.3. Differential diagnosis and imaging

ESCC main differential diagnoses are: leptomeningeal or dural metastases, intramedullary metastases or tumor, radiation myelitis and other rare causes of myelopathy such as epidural lipomatosis due to steroid administration.

The best imaging approach is MRI which if used appropriately is highly sensitive and specific. CT myelogram and standard myelography are alternate procedures of choice. Bone scan and plain radiographs are useful screening tests but are non specific and less sensitive than MRI or CT.

4.2. Headache and facial pain syndromes

Pain in the head and face is common in cancer patients. Table 7 lists the frequent and rare causes.

4.2.1. Headache due to intracranial tumor

Brain metastases have been found in 25% of the patients who die of cancer.

Headache is the most common symptom of intracranial metastases and tumors, along with mental status changes, occurring in about 50% of cases. Headache from intracranial neoplasms is due to compression or traction on pain sensitive structures (51). This process may or may not be associated with an increased intracranial pressure. It is often moderate to severe with the characteristics of tension-type headache. "Classic" brain tumor headache is associated with vomiting; it is worse in the morning and exacerbated by Valsalva and raising from bed. It can

Table 7. Differential diagnoses of new-onset headache and facial pains in cancer

Headache
1. Brain metastases
2. Skull metastases
3. Leptomeningeal metastases with altered CSF dynamics with or without hydrocephalus
4. Vascular lesion
   - Cerebral hemorrhage
     - Bleeding into metastases
     - Disseminated intravascular coagulation
     - Leukostasis
   - Cerebral infarct (usually no-headache)
     - Non-bacterial thrombotic endocarditis
     - Leukostasis
     - Superior sagittal sinus thrombosis
     - Tumor embolism
   - Subdural hematoma
   - Tumor induced subdural effusion

Facial pain
1. Facial neuralgias
   - Head and neck tumor
   - Base of the skull metastases
   - Leptomeningeal disease
2. Mucosal and cutaneous infiltration by head and neck tumors
3. Bony lesions of maxilla and mandible
4. Sinus infection
5. Lung tumor with referred facial pain

have acute exacerbations and it is more common with posterior fossa lesions and in general less common than aspecific headache.

4.2.2. Base of the skull syndromes

Base of the skull metastases are common from breast, prostate and other tumors (52) but can also result from invasion by locally advanced head and neck tumors.

Headache is felt at the site of the lesion or referred to the vertex or to the entire affected side of the head. Cranial nerve involvement together with the pain characteristics establishes a diagnosis. Table 8 reports the most common clinical findings according to the site of involvement.

4.3. Pain syndromes due to lesions of the nervous tissue

4.3.1. Facial pain due to nerve lesions

Facial neuralgia can be a manifestation of base of skull lesions or of leptomeningeal metastases but is most common from infiltration of cranial nerves by locally advanced head and neck carcinomas.

Table 8. Base of the skull syndromes causing pain

Syndrome	Pain	Cranial nerve and associated symptoms	Other symptoms and signs
Orbital	Retro-supra-orbital	II Visual loss III, IV, VI diplopia V frontal sensory loss	Chemosis, prooptosis, ipsilateral papilledema
Cavernous sinus	Supraorbital frontal	III, IV, VI diplopia V sensory loss	Papilledema
Middle cranial fossa	Trigeminal pain, can be paroxysmal Headache	VII, V, can involve cavernous sinus	
Jugular foramen	Mastoid, neck, shoulder, can be referred to the ear or pharynx	IX, X, dysphagia, XI, trapezius and sternocleidomastoid weakness XII tongue deviation	Hoarseness, Horner syndrome
Occipital condyle	Unilateral nuchal pain can radiate behind the eye Tenderness of the occipitocervical junction	XII tongue deviation	Head is tilted to avoid pain

4.3.1.1. Glossopharyngeal neuralgia

This typically produces throat and neck pain radiating to the ear and mastoid, aggravated by swallowing. This is the typical presentation of many head and neck tumors. Occasionally severe pain is associated with syncope (53). It commonly results from local nerve infiltration in the neck or base of skull (54), but it has also been described with leptomeningeal disease (55).

4.3.1.2. Trigeminal neuralgia

Middle and posterior fossa lesions can present with classic trigeminal neuralgia (56). Base of skull metastases are reviewed above. Often pain presents as a constant, dull, well localized sensation related to the underlying pathology involving bone and other somatic structures associated with paroxysmal episodes of lancinating or throbbing pain. This pattern is typical of squamous cell carcinomas of the face which often extend by perineural spread (57). Mental nerve involvement is often heralded by a paresthesia in the chin (numb chin syndrome) rarely associated with pain and is usually due to a lesion of the jaw or foramen ovale.

Table 9. Pain due to tumor involvement of nervous tissues

Mononeuropathy
–   Intercostal (most common due to chest wall tumor or metastasis)
–   Femoral
–   Obturator
–   Sciatic

Radiculopathy

Painful polyneuropathy
–   Paraneoplastic
–   Other (myeloma associated etc)

Plexopathy
–   Brachial plexopathy
–   Lumbosacral plexopathy
–   Cervical plexopathy

Cranial nerve lesion

Epidural spinal cord compression

Tumor-related headache
–   Skull lesion other than base of the skull syndromes
–   Intracranial tumor headache with or without intracranial hypertension

4.3.2. Cervical plexopathy

Tumor infiltration of the cervical plexus results from direct compression by head and neck neoplasms or from metastases to cervical nodes. Symptoms usually include local pain with lancinating or dysesthetic components referred to the retroauricular and nuchal areas, the shoulder and the jaw.

In patients who have undergone radical neck dissection followed by radiation therapy for carcinomas of the head and neck, the differential diagnosis of new onset or worsening pain due to post-treatment syndrome or tumor recurrence can be difficult. A CT scan or MRI of the neck are the appropriate imaging procedures to evaluate these problems.

4.3.3. Brachial plexopathy

Breast and lung carcinomas and lymphomas are the most common causes of brachial plexopathy. The plexus is involved by tumor in adjacent structures, such as the axillary or supraclavicular nodes, or the apex of the lung. In 85% of cases pain is the first symptom preceding other neurological symptoms or signs by weeks to months (58).

The lower plexus (C7-T1) is typically involved in both breast and lung malignancies. Pain in the shoulder, the elbow and the medial forearm with numbness in the 4th and 5th fingers is a common presentation.

In breast cancer after axillary node dissection, tumor relapse can also occur at the supraclavicular nodes. Upper plexus lesion or pan-plexopathy are more frequent in this situation. Pain is referred to the paraspinal region, shoulder, triceps region, elbow and hand. Burning dysesthesia in the index finger or the thumb is common.

Neuropathic type pain can be the prevalent symptom with numbness, paresthesias, allodynia and hyperesthesia. Pain is usually severe.

The most important differential diagnosis of a brachial plexopathy in cancer is radiation induced plexopathy. This diagnosis can be sustained by clinical, radiological and neurophysiological characteristics (59, 60).

Epidural invasion can be found in 30% of cases. It is often associated with a Horner's syndrome and pan-plexopathy (61). All patients with brachial plexopathy symptoms should have their contiguous epidural space imaged prior to being treated with radiation therapy.

4.3.4. Lumbosacral plexopathy

Lumbosacral plexopathy is frequent in pelvic malignancies. Pain is the presenting symptom in almost all cases (93%) (62) and often precedes other neurological symptoms and signs by weeks to months. It is usually followed by the onset of numbness, paresthesias, weakness and later leg edema.

The pain is initially aching or pressure-like and later becomes burning or dysesthetic.

In Jaeckle's series (62) an upper plexopathy (L1-L4) was found in about a third of cases, a lower plexopathy (L4-S1) in half of the cases and pan-plexopathy (L1-S3) in about 20%. Different levels of involvement along the plexus origin can give rise to a variety of clinical findings: selective L1 involvement, psoas muscle syndromes (L1-L3), flank pain, painful hip flexion and positive psoas muscle stretching test, sacral plexus lesions from pre-sacral masses.

Lumbosacral plexopathy often associates bone lesions to the lumbar vertebrae, sacrum, pelvis or femurs (45 of 76 patients) and epidural extension is also common. Hydroureter or hydronephrosis is extremely common at diagnosis.

Plexopathy can occur after pelvic radiation. Fundamental diagnostic criteria can be found in Thomas et al (63). Other differential diagnoses include: leptomeningeal carcinomatosis, cauda equina compression, and non cancer-related causes of lumbar plexopathy e.g. iliopsoas muscle hemorrhage or abscess, aortic aneurysm, idiopathic acute lumbosacral neuritis and post-surgical compressive lesions which often present as mononeuropathies.

Both MRI and CT scanning are the procedures of choice to image the lumbosacral plexus. The study should include L1 though the true pelvis.

4.3.5. Radiculopathies

Radiculopathies can be caused by direct invasion from a vertebral or paraspinal lesion, or by leptomeningeal metastases. Pain due to vertebral lesion is discussed above. An important cause of radicular type pain is leptomeningeal disease.

4.3.5.1. Leptomeningeal metastases (LM)

LM are due to the dissemination of neoplasm through the subarachnoid space. LM which were considered a rare complication of systemic cancer (1%–

8% of cases at autopsy) are today increasingly seen, more often due to breast, lung cancer and malignant melanoma. Prognosis is poor, reaching 3 to 6 months in intensively treated patients. Many patients are not offered treatment and their survival is shorter (64).

Headache, change in mental status and radicular type pain are the most frequent symptoms (65) but also cranial nerve involvement, seizure, polyradiculopathy and cauda equina syndrome in varying combinations are frequent presentations. Pain can be an early symptom; back pain can precede root symptom by months.

Definitive diagnosis is made with CSF examination (66), but contrast enhanced MRI can be very useful.

4.3.5.2. Herpes zoster

Other common causes of radicular pain in cancer patients are Herpes zoster and postherpetic neuralgia. Herpes zoster should always be considered in the differential diagnosis of painful radiculopathies (67).

4.3.6. Polyneuropathies

Painful polyneuropathies in cancer are usually due to chemotherapy neurotoxicity and, much more rarely, to paraneoplastic syndromes. Painful peripheral neuropathies are characterized by a stocking-glove distribution of negative (hypoesthesia) and positive sensory (burning dysesthesias, allodynia, hyperalgesia) symptoms. Vincristine, paclitaxel and paraneoplastic sensory neuropathies are typically painful, in contrast to cisplatin induced polyneuropathy which is rarely painful.

4.4. Chest wall pain

Chest wall pain is typical for lung tumors and is due to infiltration of the parietal pleura. Pain is localized with cutaneous hyperalgesia and tenderness in the overlying muscles. In a large case series of lung cancer patients, pain was unilateral in 80% of the cases and bilateral in 20% (68). Among patients with hilar tumors the pain was reported in the sternum or the scapula. In upper and lower lobe tumors, pain was referred to the shoulder and to the lower chest respectively.

Tumor progression can result in the invasion of ribs and intercostal nerves anteriorly and of vertebrae and brachial plexus superiorly and posteriorly. It is very important to recall that non-small cell lung tumors are often very aggressive and poorly responsive to oncological treatments. They cause pain syndromes that are very difficult to control and require aggressive evaluation and management.

When pain recurs after surgery, post traumatic intercostal neuropathy should be considered. However when pain persists longer than two months after thoracotomy or it recurs after a pain-free interval following surgery the probability of tumor recurrence is higher than 90% (69).

4.5. Visceral pain syndromes

In one series, visceral tumor infiltration was the second most common cause of pain in cancer patients seen at a comprehensive cancer center (70). Table 10 summarizes the most important characteristics of visceral pain syndromes and of pain arising from retroperitoneal tumors.

Table 10. Visceral pain and retroperitoneal syndromes

Syndrome	Pain characteristics
Esophageal mediastinal pain	Retrosternal, epigastric pain radiating to infrascapular region, aggravated by swallowing
Shoulder pain from diaphragmatic infiltration	
Epigastric pain from pancreatic or other upper abdominal tumor	Often radiating to the back, back pain can be the first symptom in 10–30% of cases; described as the rostral midline retroperitoneal syndrome
Adrenal metastasis or retroperitoneal distension from nodes or other tumors	Pain in the flank radiating anteriorly; described as the lateral retroperitoneal pain syndrome
Right upper quadrant pain from hepatic capsule distension	Can be referred to right scapula, shoulder and neck, acute exacerbation can occur due to bleeding of metastasis or chemoembolization. Biliary involvement can give rise to colicky pain
Diffuse abdominal pain from abdominal or peritoneal disease with or without obstruction	Pain due to peritoneal irritation can be sharp, aching and crampy. GI obstruction is a complication in 25% of ovarian cancers
Left upper quadrant pain from splenomegaly	
GI perforation	
Ureteral obstruction	
Suprapubic pain from bladder infiltration	Spasms and tenesmus
Perineal pain	See text

4.6. Pelvic and perineal pain

Gynecological, rectal and urologic tumors can cause pelvic visceral syndromes with specific patterns of referral according to the viscus involved (71).

Perineal pain, worse when sitting, with aching and pressure-like quality, that is associated with a feeling of foreign body is the first, and can be for a long time the only symptom of pelvic tumors (72). The pain results from early perineural tumor infiltration. This symptom is often associated with tenesmus (urinary or rectal according to the involvement). Prostate, cervix and rectal tumors are the most frequently associated neoplasms. Fistulas and recurrent infections can aggravate the pain syndrome. Ureteral obstruction is frequent. Direct invasion of the sacrum, sacral roots, lumbosacral plexus or cauda equina are frequent complications. These syndromes offer a good example of how visceral, somatic and neuropathic pains can be associated in advanced cancer.

5. PHARMACOLOGIC PAIN MANAGEMENT

Drug therapy can control pain in 70 to 90% of patients with chronic cancer pain, therefore pharmacologic treatment is recommended as the mainstay of chronic cancer pain management (4, 5). The WHO "analgesic ladder" (Fig. 2) can help in a sequential drug approach. This approach recommends that the analgesic drugs are selected in a stepwise fashion based on the overall severity of pain. NSAIDs are administered for mild to moderate pain. Patients with moderate to severe pain and those who fail a NSAID trial should receive an opioid conventionally used for moderate pain, usually combined with a NSAID. Severe pain or inadequate pain relief with this "second step" treatment indicates the use of an opioid conventionally used for severe pain, again possibly combined with a NSAID. Adjuvant drugs maybe added at any step to

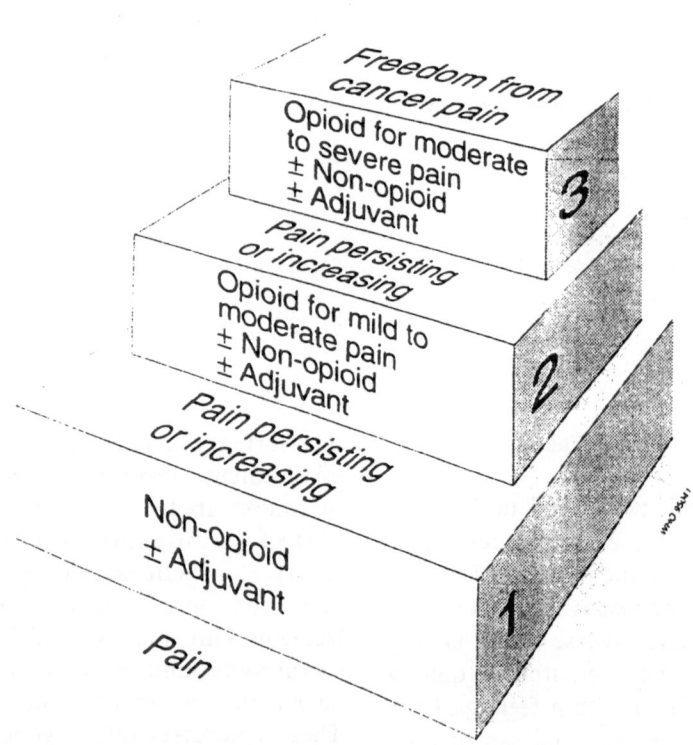

Figure 2. The three-step analgesic ladder of the World Health Organization. (Reproduced from Cancer pain relief: with a guide to opioid availability, second edition, World Health Organization, 1996, Geneva)

treat side effects or other symptoms, or as adjuvant analgesics. Recent criticism about the ladder validity (73) cannot deny that this approach closely represents common clinical practice and has greatly improved pain control if rationally applied when compared with current practice (74).

5.1. Nonsteroidal anti-inflammatory drugs

5.1.1. Analgesic effect

The NSAIDs available for pain treatment are numerous (Table 11). Their mechanism of action is mainly based on interfering with the enzyme cyclooxygenase and therefore with the production of prostaglandins. There are differences in how this mechanism operates. It is also known that NSAIDs can be analgesic through other mechanisms and finally that their action is both peripheral and central. While these complex pharmacological aspects have at the moment no impact on the clinical use of NSAIDs (75), other characteristics are of basic importance. The combination of an NSAID with an opioid produces additive analgesic effects and the combination can be useful in optimizing the balance between analgesia and side effects. NSAID efficacy is limited by a "ceiling" effect. At the ceiling, further dose increments do not yield more analgesia but can increase side effects (6, 76). This ceiling effect may help explain the limited period of time (19 days on average in one survey) (6) that these drugs can be used alone in patients who present with cancer pain.

There is no proof that any pain syndrome is more or less responsive to this class of drugs (76). Clinical experience demonstrates on the contrary, that some patients do respond electively to NSAID analgesia better than to opioid analgesia and that at times different effects can be seen with different NSAIDs, probably reflecting selectivity of action as suggested above. A comparison study showed that diclofenac, naproxen and indomethacin are all potent analgesics in cancer pain (77). NSAIDs can therefore be tried in any patient with cancer pain.

5.1.2. Toxicity

Due to advanced age, fragile medical condition, or concurrent use of other drugs, cancer patients may be relatively predisposed to toxicity from NSAIDs.

Side effects must be closely monitored during NSAID therapy, especially when using higher doses. Gastrointestinal (GI) toxicity is a particularly important concern in the elderly and in patients with a history of gastric or duodenal ulcer, requirement of higher doses, or concurrent use of corticosteroids (78). There is no relationship between dyspeptic symptoms and the development of serious GI toxicity, and two thirds of patients have no symptoms before bleeding or perforation occur. The risk of GI toxicity seems to be higher for some NSAIDs, such as ketoprofen, piroxicam and aspirin. Misoprostol administration has been associated with a decreased frequency of endoscopically detectable lesions but its efficacy in preventing the complications of long term administration is unknown (79). Co-administration of this drug is appropriate in patients who are predisposed

30

Table 11. Non-steroidal anti-inflammatory drugs

Generic name*	Half-life (h)	Starting dose (mg)†	Maximum daily dose (mg/day)	Comments
Aspirin	3–12‡	650 q 4–6 h	6000	Historical comparison. May not be tolerated as well as newer NSAIDs. Aspirin effect on platelet aggregation is non-reversible
Diflunisal	8–12	500 q 12 h	1500	Less GI toxicity than aspirin
Choline magnesium trisalicylate	8–12	1000 q 12 h	4000	Minimal GI toxicity. No effect on platelet function at usual doses
Salsalate	8–12	1000 q 12 h	4000	Minimal GI toxicity. No effect on platelet function at usual doses
Ibuprofen	3–4	400 q 6 h	4200	Metaanalyses show lowest risk of GI toxicity
Naproxen	13	225 q 12 h	1100	Greater efficacy of 1650 mg/day has been shown
Fenoprofen	2–3	200 q 6 h	3200	
Ketoprofen	2–3	25 q 6–8 h	300	
Flurbiprofen	5–6	100 q 12 h	300	
Indomethacin	4–5	50 q 8–12 h	200	Available in sustained release and rectal formulations
Sulindac	14	150 q 12 h	400	
Ketorolac	4–7	10–30 q 6 h	120	Experience limited to the treatment of acute pain. There is little experience with chronic administration
Diclofenac	2	50 q 8 h	200	
Tolmentin	1	200 q 8 h	2000	
Piroxicam	45	20 q 24 h	40	Administration at 40 mg/day over three weeks is associated with high incidence of peptic ulcer

*At high doses of any NSAID (acetaminophen is therefore excluded) stool guaiac, liver function tests, BUN, creatinine and urinalysis should be checked regularly.

†Dosing guidelines are empirical due to lack of studies on NSAIDs in the cancer population.

‡Half life of aspirin increases with dose.

to GI toxicity and those who are too frail to withstand a new GI complication. In such cases, the inability to use misoprostol should suggest empirical use of an H2 blocker, sucralfate or both.

The risk of nephrotoxicity due to NSAID therapy is higher in the elderly and those with cardiac failure, diabetes, dehydration, significant renal insufficiency and liver disease. In such patients, acetaminophen is preferred.

All NSAIDs inhibit platelet aggregation. The effect is clinically significant in patients with coagulopathies or on anticoagulant treatment; aspirin effect on platelet aggregation is very potent and non-reversible, only new platelet production will restore homeopathy.

Less common side effects include dizziness, drowsiness, cardiac failure, confusion and hypertension.

5.2. Paracetamol

Paracetamol or acetaminophen is not anti-inflammatory. Its mechanism of action is still a matter of debate, but it is probably central and is usually considered an analgesic at the same level as the NSAIDs in cancer pain management (first step of the analgesic ladder). It is an effective analgesic, especially when administered at higher doses (e.g. 1000 mg oral or IV dose/4 h) used for postoperative pain. Lower doses are included in many combinations with opioids such as codeine and oxycodone. When used alone at doses of 500 mg, it is less effective than NSAIDs. The lack of anti-inflammatory activity is probably a disadvantage in many cancer pain syndromes where peripheral inflammatory mechanisms are likely to contribute to generate pain (e.g. bone

metastases). Paracetamol has no gastric toxicity; nor does it affect platelet function. Hepatic toxicity is possible and is dose related. It is more likely in patients with alcoholism and liver disease. However 6000 mg/day is the maximally suggested daily dose and 4000 mg/day is probably a more practical end point.

5.3. Opioid analgesics

5.3.1. Basic principles

Opioid drugs can be classified according to their receptor interactions as pure agonists and agonist–antagonists (Table 12). The agonist–antagonists have a limited role in the management of chronic cancer pain due to the existence of a ceiling effect for analgesia and the potential precipitation of an abstinence syndrome in patients already physically dependent on a pure agonist drug. Several of the agonist–antagonist opioids are also more likely to produce psychomimetic effects than pure agonists (e.g. pentazocine). Agonist opioid drugs of the morphine type are the mainstay of cancer pain management.

5.3.2. "Step II" of the WHO analgesic ladder

Table 13 reports what are considered typical step II analgesic regimens.

The distinction between pure agonist opioids conventionally used for moderate pain and those used for severe pain is operational. "Weak opioid" drugs such as codeine and oxycodone are not truly weak (i.e. have no ceiling dose) but are usually given in combination with

Table 12. Opioid analgesics

Drug	10 mg IM morphine equianalgesic dose (mg)		Half life (h)	Duration (h)	Comments
	IM	PO			
Morphine-like agonists					
Morphine	10	30–60*	2–3	3–6	
Controlled release morphine		30–60		8–12	
Hydromorphone	1.5	7.5	2–3	3–4	
Oxycodone		20–30	2–3	3–6	Combined with aspirin or acetaminophen for moderate pain; available orally without coanalgesic
Oxymorphone	1	10 PR	2–3	3–4	Oral formulation not available; rectal suppositories
Meperidine	75	300	2–3	3–4	Not preferred for cancer pain due to potential toxicity
Heroin	5		0.5	4–5	Analgesic activity due to metabolites, mainly morphine
Levorphanol	2	4	12–15	3–8	Plasma accumulation occurs leading to increase in duration of clinical effects
Methadone	10**	20**	15–57	4–8	Plasma accumulation occurs leading to increase in duration of clinical effects
Ketobemidone	10	30–60	2–3	4	Available in Scandinavia No active metabolites
Codeine	130	200	2–3	3–6	Often in combination with non-opioids
Propoxyphene HCl	50	100	12	3–6	Often in combination with non-opioids
Propoxyphene napsylate	50	100	12	3–6	Often in combination with non-opioids
Hydrocodone			2–4	3–4	Available only in combination with acetaminophen
Tramadol#	100	300			
Fentanyl transdermal system	†			48–72	

Table 12. (cont)

Drug	10 mg IM morphine equianalgesic dose (mg)		Half life (h)	Duration (h)	Comments
	IM	PO			
Partial agonists					
Buprenorphine	0.3	0.8 SL	2–5	5–6	Can produce withdrawal in opioid-dependent patient; has ceiling for analgesia; sublingual tablet not available in US
Mixed agonist–antagonists					
Pentazocine	60	180	2–3	3–6	Can produce withdrawal in opioid-dependent patient; oral preparation combined with naloxone in the US; ceiling dose; psychotomimetic effects more frequent than with other opioids. Not preferred for cancer pain
Nalbuphine	10		4–6	3–6	Same profile as pentazocine, except fewer psychotomimetic effects
Butorphanol	2		2–3	3–4	Same profile as pentazocine
Dezocine	10		1.2–7.4	3–4	Same profile as pentazocine, reported to have fewer psychotomimetic effects

*Survey data suggest that the relative potency of IM to PO morphine of 1:6 changes to 1:3 with chronic dosing.

** See text for conversion to methadone and use in chronic therapy.

Tramadol is a mu receptor agonist but see text for pharmacological properties.

†Transdermal fentanyl 100 μg/h is approximately equianalgesic to morphine 4 mg/h by IV or SQ infusion, but see text for further discussion

acetaminophen or aspirin and, therefore, have a limited range of dose available. The dose of these combination products cannot exceed the maximum safe dose of the non-opioid compound (for example acetaminophen 6000 mg/day). When oxycodone and codeine are available in single preparations their dose can be increased and titrated to effects, oxycodone in particular has a favourable dose-response relationship which makes it a useful alternative to morphine or methadone (80).

Propoxyphene and meperidine have toxic metabolites that further compromise their clinical utility. At the usual doses of propoxyphene administered, this toxicity does not generally pose a clinical problem. Meperidine, however, can produce central nervous system toxicity at the parenteral doses used clinically. These effects are due to the biotransformation of meperidine to the more toxic compound, normeperidine (81). This potential of toxicity suggests that meperidine should not be used in chronic pain management.

Tramadol is a drug with opioid mu receptor agonist activity and also has monoamine reuptake blocking properties. It is used in Europe as a second step drug following the WHO ladder. This dual mechanism may allow specific indications or a lower incidence of opioid side effects at the same level of analgesia. This is partially confirmed by preliminary controlled observations showing a comparable degree of analgesia between oral tramadol and morphine with a reduction of nausea and constipation with tramadol. In this study the oral dose equivalency of tramadol with morphine was found to be 4:1. See under opioid administration for practical guidelines in managing step II opioid doses and limits.

5.3.3. Tolerance, physical dependence and addiction

A great amount of confusion among these terms on the side of physicians, nurses, patients and families contributes to preventing the correct use of opioid analgesics (11, 82, 83). To optimize opioid therapy the clinician must be ready to educate caregivers (physicians and nurses), patients and families about these issues.

Tolerance is a pharmacologic phenomenon defined by the need for escalating doses to maintain effects. Tolerance develops at different rates for the various opioid effects (84). Tolerance to respiratory depression, sedation and nausea develops rapidly, whereas tolerance to the constipating effects of opioids develops very slowly, if at all.

Tolerance to analgesic effects occurs during chronic opioid treatment (85) but is rarely a clinically significant problem. Surveys suggest the most common reason for dose escalation is worsening of pain due to tumor progression; patients with stable disease remain on stable opioid doses for very long times (86, 87). Thus tolerance is rarely an obstacle in achieving analgesia and concerns about tolerance do not justify a delay in the use of an opioid early in the course of the disease.

Physical dependence is defined by the occurrence of an abstinence syndrome after abrupt dose reduction or administration of an opioid antagonist. The dose and duration of treatment needed to develop physical dependence are not known. To be prudent, it should be assumed that any patient is physically dependent after receiving regular doses of an opioid for more than a few days.

Patients who are receiving a relatively high dose of an opioid demonstrate an increased sensitivity to antagonists. Severe withdrawal symptoms can occur after very small doses of naloxone. Given this risk, naloxone should only be used to treat symptomatic respiratory depression (see below).

Addiction is a behavioral and psychological syndrome characterized by loss of control over drug use, compulsive use and continued use despite harm. It is not a pharmacological property of opioids and should be entirely distinguished from physical dependence. Surveys show that the development of addiction in patients treated with

Table 13. Common WHO step II treatments

Codeine 30–60 mg + paracetamol 325–500 mg 1 to 2 tablets q 6–q 4.h *
Oxycodone 5–10 mg + paracetamol 325 mg 1 to 2 tablets q 6–q 4 h
Propoxyphene 90–120 + paracetamol 325 mg q 6 h
Buprenorphine 0.2 mg (sublingual tablet) 1 to 3 tablets q 8–q 6 h
Tramadol 25–200 mg q 6 h

---

* In using paracetamol combinations attention should be paid to keeping maximum daily dose ⩽4000 mg

Table 14. Drug induced alterations in opioid pharmacokinetics and/or pharmacodynamics

Opioid	Interaction	Effect
Morphine	Clomipramine	Increased bioavailability
	Amitriptyline	Increased bioavailability
Meperidine	Phenobarbital	Increased biotransformation with increased accumulation of normeperidine
	Phenytoin	Increased biotransformation with faster elimination
	Monoamine oxidase inhibitors	Excitation, hyperpyrexia, and convulsions
Methadone	Rifampin	Increased biotransformation with faster elimination
	Phenytoin	Increased biotransformation with faster elimination
Any opioids	Alcohol or other CNS depressant	Enhanced depressant effects

opioids for painful medical conditions is extremely low, and in the cancer population the occurrence of de novo addiction during pain treatment has never been reported.

5.3.4. Drug interactions and metabolic disturbances

Many drugs can modify the disposition of opioids, resulting in enhanced or decreased clinical effects. Table 13 summarizes the observations from the literature (88–93). Pharmacodynamic interactions are also common with all CNS depressant agents; such interactions could potentially produce a more pronounced sedative effect or a confusional state (94).

Multidrug treatment is very common in advanced cancer and, in most cases, there are no specific studies on pharmacokinetic or pharmacodynamic interactions. Cautious clinical judgement must be used when combining drugs in this setting.

Table 15. Oral morphine dosing guidelines

Establish initial dose	Opioid naive patient = start with 5–10 mg morphine q 4 h or equivalent
	Slow release morphine should be started at 10 mg q 12 h in most patients; higher initial dosing can be tried only with expert advice
	Patient on previous opioid regimen = see text and use conversion Table 12
Titrate dose to effect	Increase total daily dose of at least 30–50% of previous dose every 24 h until pain relief satisfactory or excessive unmanageable side effects occur
	Maximum recommended dose is immaterial, individual variability can be $\geqslant$ 10 fold
	Dose reduction may be necessary after effective alternative pain relieving procedure (e.g. RT)
Fixed dosing around the clock in accordance with the serum half life of each analgesic	In most patients with cancer it is necessary and allows pain relief and night time sleep, preventing pain reoccurrence
As needed dosing	Pain relief is often uneven and breakthrough pain is very common, always provide p.r.n. doses with a short acting opioid q 2 hours. Doses should be equal to 5-15% of daily requirements
Side effects management	Explain main side effects to the patient as potential but not unavoidable and, however, manageable
	Always give prophylactic therapy for constipation only

Metabolic disturbances must also be considered during administration of an opioid drug. Hepatic failure can modify the pharmacokinetics of some opioids. Propoxyphene, meperidine and pentazocine have longer half-lives, increased bioavailability and decreased systemic clearance in cirrhotic patients. Morphine and methadone disposition are relatively less altered by liver disease. In renal failure, metabolite accumulation should be expected with morphine, propoxyphene, meperidine and can potentially cause unexpected toxicity (95).

5.3.5. Opioid administration

5.3.5.1. First line approach

In patients with limited opioid exposure and moderate pain a combination of an opioid and non-opioid analgesic for moderate pain (step II according to the WHO ladder) is a reasonable first choice. Table 13 is non-exhaustive but can be a useful guide to clarify most common step II therapies.

In case of severe pain or of insufficient analgesia with a second step drug oral morphine should be the preferred indication (or a morphine like agonist with no limits of fast dose titration); simple guidelines which should be helpful for most cases requiring morphine administration have been laid out by an expert consensus recently (96). Table 15 summarizes the main steps to be undertaken in initiating an oral morphine regimen in patients with chronic cancer pain, and gives dosing guidelines for oral treatment in non-opioid tolerant patients.

In choosing an initial dose when patients are switched from a previous different opioid treatment, conversion tables should be used to calculate the new opioid dose. See under opioid rotation for specific recommendations (Table 12).

5.3.5.2. Routes of administration

The oral route is preferred because it is efficacious, simple and acceptable for most patients with chronic cancer pain. Alternative routes are at times made necessary due to GI tract dysfunction or the need for rapid onset or titration of analgesia. The occurrence of side effects is another potential indication for a new route. It is important to emphasize that side effects should be aggressively treated before switching either the route of administration or the drug.

Continuous infusion (subcutaneous or intravenous): The indications for continuous opioid infusion (CI) have been described in several case series (97–99) of dysphagia, GI obstruction, nausea and vomiting with oral opioids, and excessive side effects with parenteral bolus administration ("bolus effect"). CI reduces the fluctuations in plasma concentration and, for this reason, may help maintain stable plasma levels between efficacy and side effects. Subcutaneous infusion (SCI) is a very simple and effective method for implementing CI, that is also manageable in home care.

In one early study (97) it was shown that morphine SCI can be used when nausea and vomiting make oral administration impossible and also when analgesia is difficult to obtain with oral morphine or parenteral injections. Other case series substantially confirm these indications (99). The method was effective in roughly 80% of the cases in which SCI was performed in the hospital and at home. In one case series, 94% of the patients said they preferred SCI to previous therapies, whereas in another study, 16% of the patients preferred an alternative treatment because of a psychological intolerance toward infusion devices, often because of anxiety concerning having to wear and rely on an external device. Cutaneous reactions at the injection site were observed in 9% to 13% of the patients and were easily managed by changing the injection site. The tolerability of the subcutaneous needle is 7.3 ± 5.2 days (mean $\pm$ SD) and it can be improved by the use of Teflon cannulae (100).

Tolerance probably develops in all forms of opioid treatment. Portenoy and co-workers (101) described three typical patterns in opioid infusion: 1) relatively stable doses with good pain control; 2) rapidly increasing doses with good analgesia; and 3) insufficient analgesia despite the fast rate of dose increase. The last case could be the result of a relatively opioid-resistant pain syndrome (102). Doses employed vary widely across case series and largely depend on patient selection and previous opioid exposure. Different authors report average daily (SCI) dose between 65 mg (97) and 600 mg (103) morphine.

Certainly morphine is the most widely used opioid drug in SCI. Hydromorphone is widely used in the United States because of its high solubility and it is twice as potent as morphine, thus permitting a reduction in the volume of infused opioid in patients who require higher doses. Diamorphine is often preferred in Great Britain because of its high solubility. Diamorphine can help to improve local tissue compliance in cases of inflammatory reactions due to the infusion of high doses of morphine or hydromorphone, while SCI of methadone has been associated with severe local reactions (104, 105).

Controlled clinical trials comparing SCI with other forms of opioid administration are very rare. A recent double-blind cross-over study compared intravenous and subcutaneous infusion of hydromorphone for chronic cancer pain. No differences were reported in terms of side effects and analgesia. Plasma concentrations were also comparable between the two infusion methods (106). Considering the technical advantages of the subcutaneous technique, intravenous opioid infusion for severe cancer pain should be reserved for cases with specific indications such as generalized edema, coagulopathy, high frequency of local subcutaneous infection, very poor peripheral circulation (96), and in cases of severe pain when fast titration and immediate pain relief is sought.

Continuous IV infusion is however safe and feasible and can also be used in patients who have a central venous access for other therapeutic reasons. The preference of IV route for patient controlled analgesia in chronic pain is debatable.

Continuous SQ or IV infusions can be used in the home care of patients with advanced cancer to treat syndromes in which pain is associated with other symptoms such as vomiting, GI obstruction, dyspnea, agitation and delirium. An opioid (morphine and hydromorphone) can be combined with several other drugs (metoclopramide, dexamethasone, haloperidol, scopolamine, midazolam) in the same infusion (107, 108).

To set up an opioid infusion the total daily opioid consumption should be calculated and converted to parenteral morphine equivalents (using a 1:3 ratio for parenteral versus oral morphine). The resulting dose can be chosen to start the infusion and can be adapted to the situation: increased in case of poor pain control, decreased when changing the opioid drug according to guidelines for opioid rotation. In case of very limited or no previous morphine exposure the equivalent of 1–2 mg morphine per hour can be safely infused either IV or SQ providing 5 mg rescue doses p.r.n. q.1.h. The clinical context will dictate different approaches depending on pain severity and other subjective variables.

Patient-controlled analgesia: In recent years the concept of PCA gained popularity in different clinical contexts because of the wide individual variability of pain and responsiveness to analgesics. This method was successfully employed for postoperative pain often using the intravenous route. There is a wide important experience on the use of PCA for pain due to oral mucositis in bone marrow transplant chemo-radio-therapy protocols. This pain syndrome is very severe and seems to respond only partially to morphine analgesia (109). Carefully conducted studies show that perfecting PCA method of opioid infusion can be suited to patients' needs, allowing for better pain relief without increasing side effects or substantially inferior doses to obtain the same pain relief obtained from external dosing (110, 111). In this setting daily morphine doses ranged from about 40 to 80 mg in non-opioid tolerant patients.

Patient independence from staff intervention and close titration of analgesia to individual patient needs seem to constitute the main theoretical advantages of PCA for cancer pain management (112). In a cross-over study between SCI and PCA using hydromorphone for 25 patients, pain relief was comparable between the two methods; however, all patients required extra doses (mean = 6) when treated with SCI. At the end of the study, some patients preferred PCA while others preferred SCI (113).

A modified application of PCA is one in which a continuous infusion of opioids is integrated with the possibility of self administering extra boli at pre-established intervals and doses. This approach can be used very successfully with the main indication of treating breakthrough pain (103). A lock out interval of 30 to 60 minutes should be used for the SQ route and 30 minutes can be enough for the IV route. The p.r.n. dose should be equal to 15% of daily morphine equivalent requirement.

The psychological advantages of PCA have to be carefully assessed on a case-by-case basis. This system, in fact, is very useful for some patients, giving them a sense of self-control over pain and the overall situation. In other cases, the opposite is true; the responsibility of controlling one's pain and the fear of drug abuse can trigger anxiety and insecurity (114).

Spinal opioid administration: Intraspinal opioid administration is pharmacologically different from systemic administration because it can potentially yield analgesia at much lower doses. This is true however only within a very limited range of dosing in non tolerant patients. These techniques may be indicated for patients with opioid responsive pain who experience excessive side effects on systemic therapy. After epidural injection systemic redistribution of drug does occur (115), however, and some patients are unable to achieve a favorable balance between analgesia and side effects with systemic or intraspinal therapy.

Controlled clinical experiences are few. Although one study suggested that efficacy is generally comparable to oral administration (116), the likelihood of success in any individual patient is usually related to the previous systemic opioid dose (117–119). A recent survey of 1205 patients admitted to an oncology unit revealed that only 16 (1.24%) patients required spinal opioids for pain that was not controlled with systemic opioid administration, and that only six of these patients had adequate analgesia with spinal morphine alone. In the other 10 cases, analgesia was obtained only with the addition of bupivacaine to the epidural morphine (120).

A trial with a temporary catheter should always precede the implant of a chronic intraspinal system (118). Technical problems and complications related to the different catheters and infusion or access devices must be considered in selecting patients for such a trial (120). Expert follow-up is always required for management (121, 122).

Transdermal administration: The transdermal route of administration is feasible and clinically useful for the opioid fentanyl. Published clinical experience is growing with several studies showing the efficacy and safety of this approach (123-127). This route can be alternative to IV and SQ infusion in all cases of GI tract dysfunction and may be preferred to other routes of administration for reasons of patient convenience and comfort; the freedom from frequent dosing can be psychologically attractive to patients. The product can also be used when other opioids have failed due to inefficacy or bothersome side-effects (see "Opioid rotation").

Available transdermal patches can deliver 25, 50, 75 or 100 µg/h of fentanyl. It is possible to combine different patches to achieve the desired dose. Pharmacokinetic studies (126) have demonstrated large individual variability, confirming that dose titration is essential. The dosing interval for each system is 72 h. Peak plasma concentration is reached between 24 and 48 h, therefore efficacy and toxicity should generally become apparent during the first day. Dosing at 3 day intervals yields approximate steady state serum concentrations by the end of the first dose. In some patients a 48 h interval may be necessary as suggested also by pharmacokinetic data (126). After removal of the transdermal system, clinical effects will continue for many hours due to absorption of drug from a subcutaneous depot; the apparent elimination half-life is approximately 24 h.

Recent studies have suggested that transdermal fentanyl is associated with equal efficacy to oral morphine in the management of pain and a reduced incidence of constipation and nausea (127a,b,c). In a large cross-over design trial the incidence of constipation was 36.6% with oral morphine and 20.7% with transdermal fentanyl (127a). At a comparable level of pain relief patients preference favours fentanyl patch over oral morphine (both immediate and slow-release formulations).

The equianalgesic dosing of oral morphine and fentanyl patch is not fully established. The suggested ratio is 150:1 (oral morphine:fentanyl patch). In a recent study a ratio of 100:1 was used safely for patients already on oral morphine with satisfactory stable pain relief. The dose had however to be titrated upward in 58% of patients (127c) and a final conversion ratio of 70:1 was found. Table 12 reports the conversion used at a comprehensive cancer centre for patients undergoing IV morphine infusion (4 mg of morphine IV/h = 100 µg/h fentanyl patch), with previous extensive opioid exposure (R.K. Portenoy, personal communication). It is likely that this factor, previous opioid exposure, affects the

Table 16. Treatment of opioid side effects

Constipation	– Best managed with combination of cathartic and stool softener – Osmotic agents can be useful (lactulose) (enema or clysma) – Refractory constipation is exceptional can be treated with a trial of oral naloxone (see text)
Nausea–vomiting	– Alizapride metoclopramide 10 mg t.i.d – Prochlorperazine 10 mg t.i.d – Haloperidol 1–2 mg/day – Scopolamine patch – Change route of administration – Switch opioid
Sedation	– Methylphenidate 5 mg b.i.d. – Pemoline 18.75–37.50 mg b.i.d.
Delirium	– Haloperidol (neurologic/psychiatric opinion needed) – Switch opioid
Myoclonus	– Clonazepam 0.5 mg t.i.d – Switch opioid
Urinary retention	– Cholinomimetic drugs
Respiratory depression	– Naloxone; see text

differences observed in different series and also the occurrence of opioid withdrawal symptoms when changing from oral morphine to fentanyl patch.

A 100:1 ratio can be used for patients on chronic morphine therapy always providing oral or parenteral morphine rescue doses to allow flexibility of dosing especially in the first period after switching over.

Rectal route: The rectal route can be useful for treating breakthrough pain in patients who lack the oral route and are receiving transdermal fentanyl or other parenteral routes. Rectal formulations are available for morphine, oxymorphone and hydromorphone (128, 129). The bioavailability of rectal opioids is similar to oral administration and relatively erratic (129-131).

Sublingual and buccal administrations: Buprenorphine is efficacious when administered sublingually and is used in some countries for mild to moderate cancer pain (132). An oral trans-mucosal formulation of fentanyl has been developed and is under evaluation (133). It might be practical for treating breakthrough pain.

5.3.5.3. Treatment of opioid side effects

The goal of opioid therapy is a favorable balance between analgesia and side effects. The treatment of opioid side effects is, therefore, an integral part of treatment. Table 16 give practical guidelines for managing frequent and rare opioid side effects.

Constipation: It is mandatory to give

prophylactic treatment for constipation to all patients taking opioids regularly with a combination of a cathartic agent and a stool softener. There seems to be no tolerance to this effect. Oral naloxone has been used to treat refractory constipation (134, 135). This drug has a very low bioavailability (3%), and in two small case series, doses between 3 and 12 mg per day were effective without precipitating withdrawal or reversing analgesia. An initial dose of 0.8 mg once or twice a day can be carefully titrated to effect, but expert advice is suggested.

Nausea and vomiting: Significant emesis can be a problem in about 20% of patients using opioids (136). Table 16 guidelines are to be applied in a stepwise approach, eventually combining drugs with peripheral GI activity (metoclopramide, cisapride) with drugs with central antiemetic activity (metoclopramide, haloperidol, prochlorperazine). If nausea is worsened by movement or posture, scopolamine can be an option although it may exacerbate anticholinergic side effects.

Respiratory depression: is the most serious but rare opioid toxicity. The symptom is always associated with reduced level of consciousness. Tolerance to the respiratory effects of opioids develops rapidly and respiratory depression is extremely rare when opioids are carefully titrated to pain relief. The treatment of this complication with naloxone should follow very strict guidelines in the group of patients with substantial opioid exposure, because in tolerant patients even small doses of naloxone can precipitate a withdrawal syndrome. Naloxone must be diluted (1 vial, 0.4 mg in 10 ml saline) and the dose must be titrated to restore a respiratory rate of 8–12 per min. Full consciousness is not the goal of this intervention and can be achieved later with opioid tapering without putting the patient at risk of withdrawal and pain recurrence, which will occur at higher doses of naloxone. Naloxone is not recommended for oversedation without clinically significant respiratory depression. If respiratory depression occurs after slow release opioids (sustained morphine release or fentanyl patch) or methedone than the patient has to be monitored for 24 h.

5.3.5.4. Opioid rotation

Morphine is considered to be the first-line drug for severe pain, but it is now recognized that there is a wide individual variability in the response to different opioids. The therapeutic window and therefore the balance between therapeutic benefits and the pattern of adverse effects varies from drug to drug and may be more favorable with an opioid other than morphine (137, 138). This observation suggests that patients who experience dose-limiting side effects with one opioid may benefit from a trial with another opioid drug. Recent published experience shows that rotating opioid agonist drugs in case of emerging side effects with one opioid molecule without sufficient analgesia can minimize the number of patients unresponsive to opioid analgesia or experiencing severe side effects. This practice is now common in major cancer centers and palliative care units. In one series 32 of the 44 patients for whom opioids were changed due to delirium improved thereafter (139). According to preliminary experience optimizing opioid analgesia requires the availability of at least three opioids used in the management of severe pain among the following: morphine, hydromorphone, fentanyl, oxycodone, oxymorphone, methadone, levorphanol (140).

To be safe the process of switching opioid drugs requires knowledge of equianalgesic opioid dosing (Table 12). This table depicts relative potency data expressed in terms of opioid doses equianalgesic to 10 mg morphine I.M.

The information in this table is a valid starting point for all dose calculations. The dose needs to be adjusted individually and should generally be reduced by 25–50% to account for incomplete cross-tolerance between different opioids. Other factors to be considered in the size of this dose reduction are pain severity, age, metabolic abnormalities and concurrent treatments.

Half-life is another important factor that may influence the choice of an opioid and the calculation of equivalent analgesic dosing. Four to five half-lives are needed to approach a pharmacologic steady state after dosing is started or changed. Opioids with short half-lives facilitate dose titration in response to changes in pain intensity and are preferred when rapid dose titration is needed, specifically when pain is very severe. The half-life of methadone ranges from 12 to more than 100 h; delayed toxicity due to accumulation is possible after initiating therapy or increasing the dose (141, 142).

In switching patients from hydromorphone to methadone the ratio which was found effective clinically was 1.2 ± 1.3 for methadone/hydromorphone oral doses (143) instead of the expected ratio of 5-7 based on the single dose available data. This depends most likely on the accumulation kinetics achieved with repeated dosing. When

converting any opioid to methadone, a reduction of the equivalent dose by at least 75% is suggested.

5.4. Opioid resistant pain

In case of pain syndromes with poor response to opioids it is difficult to determine whether pain is in fact unresponsive to opioid analgesics or if the dose–effect slope is so moved to the right in some cases as to make opioid treatment impractical due to the onset of undesired side effects (102). It is true that most cases of unresponsive opioid pain can be managed by appropriate upward titration, possibly by changing the administration from oral to parenteral in cases of excessive gastrointestinal side effects at high oral doses. Nevertheless in some pain syndromes there is an unfavorable response to opioid therapy. Neuropathic pain with a major deafferentation component is considered to be usually relatively resistant to opioids. Perineal pain with rectal and vesical tenesmus and mucosal burning pain, such as in post-chemo-radio-therapy mucositis, are other examples (109). A working definition might be useful in clinical practice: an opioid resistant pain syndrome should imply either no response or an insufficient analgesic response despite an upward titration of full agonist opioids through a reliable administration route (the best choice would be intravenous infusion) to the point of unacceptable central nervous system side effects (102). In a recent study, neuropathic pain showed a relative resistance to opioids, but 50% of the pain syndrome diagnosed as neuropathic did show a response (144). In another study, the presence of plexus or nerve involvement had no negative impact on pain relief, whereas only 6% of the patients with bone metastasis were pain-free when moving (145).

As already mentioned in the study by Hogan and co-workers (120) 1.24% of cancer patients were reported to be unmanageable with systemic opioids, and 75% of them with neuropathic pain required bupivacaine spinal infusion to achieve analgesia. A report by Du Pen and co-workers (146) presenting a case series of 375 patients covering 5 years of activity shows that 18% failed to respond to aggressive epidural opioid escalation, and 90% of the non responders could be managed with a combination of morphine and bupivacaine. Postural hypotension was observed in 9% of the cases. No central nervous system or systemic toxicity was reported. Similar results have been reported on the use of intrathecal bupivacaine and morphine with a higher incidence of urinary retention (24%) (147). With selected patients, pain pathway blocks can be considered as an alternative to continuous anesthetic blockade when nociceptive pain is implicated; adjuvant analgesics should be tried in all patients with opioid resistant neuropathic pain.

5.5 Adjuvant analgesics

Some of these drugs have primary indications other than analgesia, but are analgesics in selected circumstances and pain syndromes for which they are given as primary pain therapy (e.g. tricyclic antidepressants for postherpetic neuralgia or carbamazepine for trigeminal neuralgia). Cancer pain can have complex pathophysiologies and is usually responsive to opioid analgesia. An ad-

juvant analgesic can help improving pain relief in specific indications (Table 17).

5.5.1. Tricyclic antidepressants

The analgesic effect of tricyclic antidepressants has been proven in typical neuropathic pain syndromes such as diabetic neuropathy and postherpetic neuralgia (148, 149). The dissociation of the analgesic effect from the antidepressant effect has been clearly demonstrated (150). The analgesic effect is seen much earlier than antidepressant effects. Amitriptyline is sometimes preferred due to its useful hypnotic effects. The effective dose range is the same across different drugs and is usually between 50 mg and 150 mg/day in one or two daily doses. But doses as low as 25 mg/day can be effective Desipramine and nortriptyline have less sedating and anticholinergic side effects and may be preferred in some patients on this basis. The pharmacokinetic interaction of tricyclics with morphine should always be kept in mind (Table 13).

There is no clinical indication for using non-tricyclic antidepressants as adjuvant analgesics.

5.5.2. Anticonvulsants and baclofen

The analgesic effect of the anticonvulsants carbamazepine and phenytoin is well established in trigeminal neuralgia (151). Anticonvulsants are especially useful in cancer pain with lancinating or paroxysmal dysesthesias (152). Carbamazepine is preferred because of the wider clinical experience with this drug, but the marrow toxicity from this drug limits its utility in those patients receiving myelosuppressive therapy. Usual

Table 17. Adjuvant drugs for neuropathic cancer pain

Class	Drug	Notes
Tricyclic antidepressants	Amitriptyline Imipramine Desimipramine Nortriptyline	Burning dysesthetic pain
Anticonvulsants	Carbamazepine Phenytoin Sodium valproate Clonazepam	Lancinating paroxysmal pain
Central GABAergic	Baclofen	Lancinating paroxysmal pain
Oral local anesthetics	Tocainamide Mexiletine	
Steroids	Dexamethasone methylprednisolone	For nerve compression pain, suggestive evidence
α_2-Adrenergic antagonists	Clonidine	Epidural use: orthostatic hypotension main limit, transdermal patch: preliminary data
NMDA receptor antagonists	Ketamine Dextromethorphan	Evidence is preliminary, not recommended in clinical practice

doses of carbamazepine can range between 400 and 1600 mg/day. Other anticonvulsants such as valproate and clonazepam have been less studied for neuropathic pain and their efficacy is not proven. Baclofen, which is not an anticonvulsant, also has proven efficacy in trigeminal neuralgia (153) and, on this basis, is sometimes used for paroxysmal or lancinating neuropathic pains. The list of anticonvulsants in Table 17 reflects our opinion on their relative indication (top to bottom in the list) of these drugs for lancinating neuropathic pain and is based on the literature results and on personal experience.

5.5.3. Corticosteroids

The wide use of steroids in advanced cancer is not always justified (154). They have efficacy in relieving pain and improving appetite, nausea, mood and overall quality of life in this patient population (155) but their effect should be carefully monitored and they should be tapered to minimum useful dose or stopped when possible. In some painful conditions, such as raised intracranial pressure, spinal cord compression, superior vena cava syndrome, metastatic bone pain, nerve plexus or peripheral nerve compression, symptomatic lymphedema and hepatic capsular distension, the administration of an IV bolus of dexamethasone (10 to 100 mg)

(156, 157) or methylprednisolone (50 to 250 mg) (personal experience) can have dramatic analgesic effects.

5.5.4. Oral local anesthetic

Neuropathic pain may respond to IV lidocaine infusion (158) and, recently, the efficacy of oral tocainide and mexiletine has been similarly documented for painful diabetic neuropathy (159) and nerve injury pain (160). A trial with oral mexiletine can be recommended in neuropathic pain syndromes failing to respond to the use of antidepressants starting with 150–200 mg once a day and increasing by one dose unit every three to five days (149). Most common side effects are nausea and heartburn which can be anticipated by taking the drug with food. Other more rare side effects are sedation, dizziness and tremors. Toxic blood levels can produce seizures. Mexiletine is contraindicated in patients with second or third degree atrioventricular blockade. Common daily doses are around 10 mg/kg. A small case series also reported the efficacy of subcutaneous lidocaine infusion in neuropathic cancer pain (161).

5.5.5. Adjuvants used in the treatment of bowel obstruction

Bowel obstruction is a fairly frequent complication of advanced abdominal cancer. When this clinical condition is not surgically reversible, the management of pain and associated symptoms (mainly vomiting) can be accomplished using drugs, typically administered by continuous SQ or IV infusions. Anticholinergic drugs, like scopolamine and glycopyrrolate, have been effective in reducing colicky pain and vomiting

(162). More recently, octreotide, a synthetic analogue of somatostatin, has been proven effective in reducing or eliminating vomiting in patients with bowel obstruction (163).

5.5.6. Bisphosphonates for bone pain

Bisphosphonates inhibit osteoclastic activity and are effective in the treatment of cancer-associated hypercalcemia. Due to their poor oral bioavailability, they are generally given IV initially although clodronate is available in capsules. Clodronate and pamidronate are the main representatives of this class of drugs used in clinical practice. Both have been used in the long-term care of patients with bone disease and pain. In placebo controlled studies both clodronate and pamidronate reduced the incidence of bone metastases related complications and improved pain relief (164). An advantage in terms of relief of bone pain can be found in about 30–50% of patients treated with clodronate IV. Pamidronate disodium is a more potent inhibitor of bone resorption at doses that do not affect bone mineralization. Its analgesic activity seems to be dose-dependent (165, 166), with about 60% of patients reporting relevant pain reduction with 60 and 90 mg 4-weekly regimens.

Recent data suggest that at least in multiple myeloma the early prophylactic use of pamidronate could be recommended to reduce the complications related to bone disease including pain, fractures and spinal cord compression (167). These potential guidelines need further validation but a trial of pamidronate can be recommended in refractory bone pain. Doses of 90 mg IV seem more effective than 60 mg and a 3 weekly course regimen is usually well tolerated. An alternative could be clodronate at 600 mg IV daily for a few days. If pain relief is reached, a maintenance treatment with oral clodronate is recommended. The cost of these agents should however be considered, based on the coming literature, when planning treatment.

6. INVASIVE TECHNIQUES FOR PAIN MANAGEMENT

Available data on the implementation of the WHO "analgesic ladder" suggest that about 20–30% of patients with cancer pain do not achieve a satisfactory balance between pain relief and side effects using drugs alone via the common routes. It is not known how many of this group will benefit from spinal opioids and local anesthetic. Anesthetic and neurosurgical techniques in a selected group may reduce the requirements for systemic drugs to achieve adequate analgesia.

Nerve blocking or neurolytic procedures have been widely used in the past. In cancer pain their use has greatly diminished after the widespread introduction of pharmacotherapy (168). All these techniques require considerable skills and expertise to be safely performed and therefore they should be reserved for highly specialized centers. Pain syndrome indication is fundamental and an open discussion with the patient of potential side effects is also essential (169). It is also important to

Table 18. Invasive techniques available for cancer pain management

Procedure	Indication	Complications	Notes
Neurolytic subarachnoid blockade	Localized pain Short prognosis Perineal pain with previous sphincter impairment	Dysesthesia Motor-sensory disturbance Sphincter impairment	Skilled performer will minimize complications
Celiac plexus block	Visceral pain from upper abdominal viscera (e.g. pancreas)	Orthostatic hypotension Myelopathy-paraplegia	Usually transitory Extremely rare
Hypogastric plexus block	Visceral pelvic pain	?	Clinical experience limited
Trigeminal ganglion block	Head and neck cancer pain in trigeminal distribution	Corneal anesthesia	Several techniques available
Cervical percutaneous cordotomy	Unilateral pain	Homolateral leg weakness Sphincter disturbances Orthostatic hypotension Impotence Respiratory failure	Transitory frequent, permanent deficit rare All complications are more frequent with bilateral procedure See text See text

make clear that the analgesic effect can be partial or temporary and that most patients will require complementary pharmacotherapy for pain control either immediately or later on (170, 171). Whether the potential drug sparing effect of these interventions is beneficial or not is debatable (172). It is now generally accepted that invasive procedures should be reserved after rational pharmacological treatment, including the failed use of spinal catheter therapy (173, 174).

Table 18 lists the procedures, main indications and complications. This list is not exhaustive but includes all the procedures which we can consider feasible and useful in selected indications in cancer patients.

6.1. Neurolytic blockades

6.1.1. Celiac plexus block

The best indication for the celiac plexus block is upper abdominal visceral pain due to pancreatic involvement or to neoplastic spreading on the celiac axis after failure of analgesic drug titration (175). The technique currently in use allows the celiac plexus region to be located percutaneously, and subsequently a neurolytic substance (phenol or alcohol) is injected. Alcohol is preferred because it is less toxic to tissues and vasal structures. Duration and completeness of analgesia is unpredictable also for pain with celiac characteristics. Pain management needs usually to be integrated with drug therapy, in fact, roughly 16% of the patients obtained complete pain relief until death in one study (171). Studies comparing

pharmacological therapies with CPB are rare and the number of patients are very small, but they seem to confirm that analgesia appears to lean in favour of the celiac block during the first weeks after treatment. This advantage is no longer present after two to four weeks (172,175a,b). An analgesic drug sparing effect has also been observed and might be useful in reducing drug-related side-effects (172, 175a). Orthostatique hypotension and transient diarrhoea are the most common side-effects, found in nearly 30% to 60% of the cases, and, therefore, measures should be taken to prevent or treat them. Side-effects having a lesser impact on the patient are transient dysesthesia, reactive pleurisy, and transient hematuria due to renal puncture. Some rare, though serious, side-effects have been described, among them are peripheral neurologic lesions (due to alcohol injections into the psoas muscle or at the lumbar plexus level) or central neurologic lesions such as paraplegia (probably due to medullary ischemia from damage to the Adamkiewicz artery) (175c).

6.1.2. Subarachnoid neurolytic blocks

The administration of chemical agents into the epidural or intrathecal space was once a very common treatment for cancer pain. In our opinion, the spinal injection of either hypobaric alcohol solution or hyperbaric phenol in glycerin has no selective action on sensitive pain fibres. There is, therefore, a high risk of disabling lesions. We will limit our descriptions to the cauda-equina rhizotomy technique, as it is the only one we perform for perineal pain. With the patient in seated position, a 23-guage needle is introduced through L5–

50

S1 interspace into the subarachnoid space. An 0.8-ml solution of 7.5% phenol in glycerin is then slowly injected. The patient is kept in this position for 30 min. We use chemical rhizotomy when a patient suffering from perineal pain shows clear signs of somatic pain, disease recurrence, macroscopic areas of vulvovaginal or pararectal erosion, evident 'trigger points', problems with micturition due to a pre-existing bladder dysfunction and already have a colostomy. Our experience on 39 patients with perineal pain treated with chemical rhizotomy shows average duration of pain relief of 5.4 months (175d). Bladder sphincter complications were noted in 19 patients (49%). Problems concerning anal sphincter dysfunction did not develop in our patients mainly because 79% of them had submitted to colostomy beforehand.

6.2. Neuroablative techniques

6.2.1. Cervical percutaneous cordotomy

Percutaneous cordotomy is the most efficacious of these techniques. Due to its selectivity on the spinothalamic tract of the spinal cord this technique produces complete analgesia on the contralateral hemibody including C5-S5 dermatomes. It is a very difficult procedure, especially when a high dermatomal level of analgesia is required. In expert hands the rate of persistent complication is limited to 1% mortality, 5% bladder dysfunction, and 8-20% homolateral leg weakness (168–177). It is performed under local anesthesia and poses a considerable burden on the patient, who has to be cooperative. It is very important that the patient prognosis does not outlast 1 year due to the risk of developing post cordotomy dysesthetic pain which is also the main reason for not performing cordotomies for benign pain. The incidence of complications is higher with bilateral cordotomy and this procedure is not recommended (177).

REFERENCES

1. Greenwald H. P., Bonica J. J., Bergner M.: The prevalence of pain in four cancers. Cancer 60: 2563–9, 1987
2. Portenoy R. K., Miransky J., Thaler H. T., Hornung J., Bianchi C., Cibas-Kong I., Feldhamer E., Lewis F., Matamoros I., Sugar M. Z., Olivieri A. P., Kemeny N. E., Foley K. M.: Pain in ambulatory patients with lung and colon cancer. Prevalence, characteristics, and effect. Cancer 70: 1616–24, 1992
3. Portenoy R. K., Kornblith A. B., Wong G., Vlamis V., McCarthy Lepore J., Loseth D. B., Hakes T., Foley K. M., Hoskins W. J.: Pain in ovarian cancer patients. Prevalence, characteristics, and associated symptoms. Cancer 74: 907–15, 1994
4. Jacox A., Carr D. B., R. P. et al.: Management of cancer pain. Clinical practice guideline N. 9. AHCPR Publication N 94-0592. Rockville MD: Agency for Health Care Policy and Research, U.S. Department of Health and Human Services, Public Health Service, 1994
5. World Health Organization. Cancer Pain Relief. 2nd edition. Geneva: World Health Organization, 1996
6. Ventafridda V., Tamburini M., Caraceni A., DeConno F., Naldi F.: A validation study of the WHO method for cancer pain relief. Cancer 59: 851–6, 1987
7. Cleeland C. S., Gonin R., Hatfield A. K., Edmonson J. H., Blum R. H., Stewart J. A., Pandya K. J.: Pain and its treatment in outpatients with metastatic cancer. N Engl J Med 330: 592–6, 1994
8. Larue F., Colleau S. M., Brasseur L., Cleeland C. S.: Multicentre study of cancer pain and its management in France. Br Med J 310: 1034–7, 1995
9. Von Roenn J. H., Cleeland C. S., Gonin R., Hatfield A., Pandya K. J.: Physician's attitudes and practice in cancer pain management: A survey from the Eastern Cooperative Oncology Group. Ann Intern Med 119: 121–6, 1993
10. Larue F., Colleau S. M., Fontaine A., Brasseur L.: Oncologists and primary care physicians' attitudes toward pain control and morphine prescribing in France. Cancer 76: 2375–82, 1995
11. Ward S. E., Goldberg N., Miller-McCauley V., Mueller C., Nolan A., Pawlik-Plank D., Robbins A., Stormoen D., Weissman D. E.: Patient related barriers to management of cancer pain. Pain 52: 319–24, 1993
12. Zech D. F. J., Grond S., Lynch J., Hertel D., Lehman K. A.: Validation of World Health Organization guidelines for cancer pain relief. A 10-year prospective study. Pain 63: 65–76, 1995
13. Grond S., Zech D., Diefenbach C., Radbruch L., Lehman K. A.: Assessment of cancer pain: a prospective evaluation in 2266 cancer patients referred to a pain service. Pain 64: 107–14, 1996
14. Portenoy R. K., Hagen N. A.: Breakthrough pain: definition, prevalence and characteristics. Pain 41: 273–81, 1990
15. Gonzales G. R., Elliot K. J., Portenoy R. K., Foley K. M.: The impact of a comprehensive evaluation in the management of cancer pain. Pain 47: 141–4, 1991
16. Au E., Loprinzi C. L., Dhodapkar M., al. e.: Regular use of verbal pain scale improves the understanding of oncology inpatient pain intensity. J Clin Oncol 12: 2751–5, 1994
17. Jensen M. P., Karoly K.: Measurement of cancer pain by self report. In: Chapman, C. R. and Foley, K. M. (eds): Current and Emerging Issues in Cancer Pain: Research and Practice, Raven Press, New York, 1993, pp 193–218
18. Serlin R. C., Mendoza T. R., Nakamura Y., Edwards K. R., Cleeland C. S.: When is cancer pain mild, moderate or severe? Grading pain severity by its interference with function. Pain 61: 277–84, 1995
19. Melzack R., Casey K. L.: Sensory, motivational and central control determinants of pain: a new conceptual model. In: Kenshalo, D. (ed.): The skin senses, CC Thomas, Springfield, IL, 1968, pp 423–39
20. Melzack R.: The McGill pain questionnaire: Major properties and scoring methods. Pain 1: 277–99, 1975
21. Daut R. L., Cleeland C. S., Flanery R. C.: Development of the Wisconsin Brief Pain

Questionnaire to assess pain in cancer and other diseases. Pain 17: 197–210, 1983

22. Fishman B., Pasternak S., Wallenstein S. L., Houde R. W., Holland J. C., Foley K. M.: The Memorial Pain Assessment Card: A valid instrument for the evaluation of cancer pain. Cancer 60: 1151–8, 1987

23. De Conno F., Caraceni A., Gamba A., Mariani L., Abbatista A., Brunelli C., La Mura A., Ventafridda V.: Pain measurement in cancer patients: a comparison of six methods. Pain 57: 161–6, 1994

24. Greenwald H. P.: Interethnic differences in pain perception. Pain 44: 157–63, 1991

25. Caraceni A., Mendoza T., Mencaglia E., Baratella C., Edwards K., Forjaz M., Martini C., Serlin R., De Conno F., Cleeland C.: A validation study of the Italian version of the Brief Pain Inventory (Breve Questionario per la Valutazione del Dolore). Pain 65:87–92, 1996

26. Daut R. L., Cleeland C. S.: The prevalence and severity of pain in cancer. Cancer 50: 1913–18, 1982

27. Ventafridda V., De Conno F., Di Trapani P., et al.: A new method of pain quantification based on weekly self–descriptive record of intensity and duration of pain. In: Bonica, J. J., Lindblom, U., Iggo, A. et al. (eds): Advances in Pain Research and Therapy vol. 6, Raven Press, New York, 1983, pp 892–5

28. Ingham J. M., Portenoy R. K.: Symptom Assessment. Hematol Oncol Clin N Am 10: 57–78, 1996

29. American Pain Society Quality of Care Committee: Quality improvement guidelines for the treatment of acute pain and cancer pain. J Am Med Assoc 274: 1874–80, 1995

30. Foley K. M.: Pain syndromes in patients with cancer. In: Bonica, J. J. and Ventafridda, V. (eds): Advances in Pain Research and Therapy, vol.2, Raven Press, New York, 1979, pp 59–75

31. Portenoy R. K.: Cancer pain: pathophysiology and syndromes. Lancet 339: 1026–31, 1992

32. Arner S., Arner B.: Differential effect of epidural morphine in the treatment of cancer-related pain. Acta Anaesthesiol Scand 29: 32–6, 1985

33. Rowbotham M. C., Reisner L., Fields H. L.: Both intravenous lidocaine and morphine reduce the pain of postherpetic neuralgia. Neurology 41: 1024–8, 1991

34. McQuay H. J., Jadad A. R., Carroll D., Faura C., Glynn C. J., Moore R. A., Liu Y.: Opioid sensitivity of chronic pain: a patient-controlled analgesia method. Anaesthesia 47: 757–67, 1992

35. Cherny N. I., Thaler H. T., Friedlander-Klar H., Lapin J., Foley K. M., Houde R., Portenoy R. K.: Opioid responsiveness of cancer pain syndromes caused by neuropathic or nociceptive mechanisms: A combined analysis of controlled single dose studies. Neurology 44: 857–61, 1994

36. Ventafridda V., Caraceni A.: Cancer pain classification: a controversial issue. Pain 46: 1–2, 1991

37. Tasker R.: Management of nociceptive, de-afferentation, and central pain by surgical intervention. In: Fields, H. L. (ed.): Pain Syndromes in Neurology, Butterworths, London, 1990, pp 143–200

38. Cherny N. I., Portenoy R. K.: Cancer Pain: principles of assessment and syndromes. In: Wall, P. D. and Melzack, R. (eds): Textbook of Pain, Churchill Livingstone, Edinburgh, 1994, pp 787–823

39. Caraceni A.: Clinicopathological correlates of common cancer pain syndromes. Hematol Oncol Clin N Am 10: 57–78, 1996

40. Healey J.: The mechanism and treatment of bone pain. In: Arbit, E. (ed.): Management of cancer-related pain, Futura, New York, 1993, pp 515–26

41. Hacking H. G., Van A. H., Lankhorst G. J.: Factors related to the outcome of inpatient rehabilitation in patients with neoplastic epidural spinal cord compression. Paraplegia 31: 367–74, 1993

42. Portenoy R. K., Lipton R. B., Foley K. M.: Back pain in the cancer patient: an algorithm for evaluation and management. Neurology 37: 134–8, 1987

43. Posner J. B.: Back pain and epidural spinal cord compression. Med Clin N Am 71: 185–206, 1987

44. Ventafridda V., Caraceni A., Martini C., Sbanotto A., De C. F.: On the significance of Lhermitte's sign in oncology. J Neuro-oncol 10: 133–7, 1991

45. Rodichok L. D., Harper G. R., Ruckdeschel J. C., et al: Early diagnosis of spinal epidural metastases. Am J Med 70: 1181–8, 1981

46. Rodichok L. D., Ruckdeschel J. C., Harper G. R., et al.: Early detection and treatment of spinal epidural metastases: the role of myelography. Ann Neurol 20: 696, 1986

47. Portenoy R. K., Galer B. S., Salamon O., Freilich M., Finkel J. E., Milstein D., Thaler H. T., Berger M., Lipton R. B.: Identification of epidural neoplasm. Radiography and bone scintigraphy in the symptomatic and asymptomatic spine. Cancer 64: 2207–13, 1989

48. Graus F., Krol G., Foley K. M.: Early diagnosis of spinal epidural metastasis: Correlation with clinical and radiological findings. Proceedings of the American Society of Clinical Oncology 5: Abstract 1047, 1986

49. Haddad P., Thaell J. F., Kiely J. M., Harrison E. G., Miller R. H.: Lymphoma of the spinal epidural space. Cancer 38: 1862–6, 1976

50. Lewis D. W., Packer R. J., Raney B.: Incidence, presentation and outcome of spinal cord disease in children with systemic cancer. Pediatrics 78: 438, 1986

51. Forsyth P. A., Posner J. B.: Intracranial neoplasm. In: Olesen, J., Tfelt–Hansen, P. and Welch, K. M. A. (eds): The Headaches, Raven Press, New York, 1993, pp 705–14

52. Greenberg H. S., Deck M. D. F., Vikram B., et al: Metastasis to the base of the skull: Clinical findings in 43 patients. Neurology 31: 530–7, 1981

53. Weinstein R. E., Herec D., Friedman J. H.: Hypotension due to glossopharyngeal neuralgia. Arch Neurol 40: 90–2, 1986

54. Vecht C. J., Hoff A. M., Kansen P. J., de B. M., Bosch D. A.: Types and causes of pain in cancer of the head and neck. Cancer 70: 178–84, 1992

55. Sozzi C., Marotta P., Piatti L.: Vagoglossopharyngeal neuralgia with syncope in the course of carcinomatous meningitis. Ital J Neurol Sci 8: 271–6, 1987

56. Cheng T. M., Cascino T. L., Onofrio B. M.: Comprehensive study of diagnosis and treatment of trigeminal neuralgia secondary to tumors. Neurology 43: 2298–302, 1993

57. Carter R. L., Pittam M. R., Tanner N. S. B.: Pain and dysphagia in patients with squamous carcinomas of the head and neck: the role of perineural spread. J R Soc Med 75: 598–606, 1982

58. Kori S. H., Foley K. M., Posner J. B., et al: Brachial plexus lesions in patients with cancer: 100 cases. Neurology 31: 45–50, 1981

59. Lederman R. J., Wilbourn A. J.: Brachial plexopathy: Recurrent cancer or radiation? Neurology 34: 1331–5, 1984

60. Foley K.: Brachial plexopathy in patients with breast cancer. In: Harris, J. R., Hellman, S., Henderson, I. C. and Kinne, D. (eds): Breast Diseases, Lippincott, Philadelphia, 1991, pp 722–9

61. Cascino T. L., Kori S., Krol G., Foley K. M.: CT scan of brachial plexus in patients with cancer. Neurology 33: 1553–7, 1983

62. Jaeckle K. A., Young D. F., Foley K. M.: The natural history of lumbosacral plexopathy in cancer. Neurology 35: 8–15, 1985

63. Thomas J. E., Cascino T. L., Earl J. D.: Differential diagnosis between radiation and tumor plexopathy of the pelvis. Neurology 35: 1–7, 1985

64. Siegal T., Lossos A., Pfeffer M. R.: Leptomeningeal metastases. Analysis of 31 patients with sustained off-therapy response following combined-modality therapy. Neurology 44: 1463–1469, 1994

65. Kaplan J. G., DeSouza T. G., Farkash A., Shafran B., Pack D., Rehman F., Fuks J., Portenoy R.: Leptomeningeal metastases: comparison of clinical features and laboratory data of solid tumors, lymphomas and leukemias. J Neurooncol 9: 225–9, 1990

66. Wasserstrom W. R., Glass J. P., Posner J. B.: Diagnosis and treatment of leptomeningeal metastasis from solid tumors: Experience with 90 patients. Cancer 49: 759–72, 1982

67. Rowbotham M. C.: Postherpetic neuralgia. Semin Neurol 14: 247–54, 1994

68. Marino C., Zoppi M., Morelli F., Buoncristiano U., Pagni E.: Pain in early cancer of the lungs. Pain 27: 57–62, 1986

69. Kanner R., Martini N., Foley K. M.: Nature and incidence of postthoracotomy pain. Proceedings of the American Society of Clinical Oncology 1: Abstract 590, 1982

70. Martini C.: Sindromi dolorose da Cancro. Univerita' degli Studi di Milano, Facolta' di Medicina a Chirurgia, Scuola di Specializzazione in Oncologia, 1991

71. Stillman M.: Perineal pain: Diagnosis and management, with particular attention to perineal pain of cancer. In: Foley, K. M., Bonica, J. J. and Ventafrida, V. (eds): Second

international congress on cancer pain, 16, Raven Press, New York, 1990, pp 359–77

72. Boas R. A., Schug S. A., Acland R. H.: Perineal pain after rectal amputation: a 5-year follow-up. Pain 52: 67–70, 1993

73. Jadad A. R., Browman G. P.: The WHO analgesic ladder for cancer pain management. Stepping up the quality of its evaluation. J Am Med Assoc 274: 1870–3, 1995

74. Ventafridda V., Caraceni A., Gamba A.: Field-testing of the WHO guidelines for cancer pain relief. In: Foley, K. M., Ventafridda, V. and Bonica, J. J. (eds): Advances in Pain Research and Therapy, vol. 16. 2nd International Congress on Cancer Pain, Raven Press, New York, 1990, pp 451–64

75. Brookes P. M., Day R. O.: Non–steroidal antiinflammatory drugs: differences and similarities. N Engl J Med 324: 1716–25, 1991

76. Eisenberg E., Berkey C. S., Carr D. B., Mostseller F., Chalmers T. C.: Efficacy and safety of nonsteroidal antiinflammatory drugs for cancer pain: a metaanalysis. J Clin Oncol 12: 2756–65, 1994

77. Ventafridda V., De Conno F., Panerai A. E., Maresca V., Monza G. C., Ripamonti C.: Non-steroidal anti-inflammatory drugs as the first step in cancer pain therapy: double-blind, within-patient study comparing nine drugs. J Int Med Res 18: 21–9, 1990

78. Loeb D. S., Ahlquist D. A., Talley N. J.: Management of gastroduodenopathy associated with use of nonsteroidal anti-inflammatory drugs. Mayo Clin Proc 67: 354–64, 1992

79. Ingham J. M., Portenoy R. K.: Drugs in the treatment of pain: NSAIDS and Opioids. Curr Opin Anaethesiol 6: 838–44, 1993

80. Kalso E., Vainio A.: Morphine and oxycodone hydrochloride in the management of cancer pain. Clin Pharmacol Ther 47: 639–46, 1990

81. Kaiko R. F., Foley K. M., Grabinski P. V., Heidrich G., Rogers A. G., Inturrisi C. E., Reidenberg M. M.: Central nervous system excitatory effects of meperidine in cancer patients. Ann Neurol 13: 180–5, 1983

82. Warncke T., Breivik H., Vainio A.: Treatment of cancer pain in Norway. A questionnaire study. Pain 57: 109–16, 1994

83. Vortherms R., Ryan P., Ward S.: Knowledge of, attitudes toward, and barriers to pharmacologic management of cancer pain in a statewide random sample of nurses. Res Nurs Health 15: 459–66, 1992

84. Portenoy R. K.: Tolerance to opioid analgesics: clinical aspects. In: Hanks, G.W. (ed.): Cancer Surveys Volume 21: Palliative Medicine: Problem Areas in Pain and Symptom Management, 1994, pp 49–65

85. Foley K. M.: Clinical tolerance to opioids. In: Basbaum, A. I. and Bessom, J. M. (eds): Towards a New Pharmacotherapy of Pain, Dahlem Konfrenzen., John Wiley & Sons, Chichester, 1991, pp 181–204

86. Twycross R. G.: The use of narcotic analgesics in terminal illness. J Med Ethics 1: 10–17, 1975

87. Kanner R. M., Foley K. M.: Patterns of narcotic drug use in a cancer pain clinic. Ann NY Acad Sci 362: 161–72, 1981

88. Inturrisi C. E.: Effects of other drugs and pathologic states on opioid disposition and response. In: Benedetti, C., Giron, G. and Chapman, C. R. (eds): Raven Press, New York, 1990, pp 171–81

89. Ventafridda V., Ripamonti C., DeConno F., Bianchi M., Pazzuconi F., Panerai A. E.: Antidepressants increase bioavailability of morphine in cancer patients (letter). Lancet 1: 1204, 1987

90. Stambaugh J. E., Hemphill D. M., Wainer I. W., Schwartz I.: A potentially toxic drug interaction between pethidine (meperidine) and phenobarbitone. Lancet 1: 398–9, 1977

91. Pond S. M., Kretschzma K. M.: Effect of phenytoin on meperidine clearance and normeperidine formation. Clin Pharmacol Ther 30: 680–6, 1981

92. Kreek M. J., Garfield J. W., Gutjahr C. L., Giusti, L.M.: Rifampin-induced methadone withdrawal. N Engl J Med 294: 1104–6, 1976

93. Tong T. G., Pond, S.M., Kreek M. J., Jaffery N. F., Benowitz N. L.: Phenytoin-induced methadone withdrawal. Ann Intern Med 94: 349–51, 1981

94. Caraceni A., Martini C., De Conno F., Ventafridda V.: Organic brain syndromes and opioid administration for cancer pain. J Pain Symptom Manage 9: 527–33, 1994

95. Bortolussi R., Fabiani F., Savron F., Testa V., Lazzarini R., Sorio R., De Conno F., Caraceni A.: Acute morphine intoxication during high-dose recombinant Interleukin-2 treatment for metastatic renal cell cancer. Eur J Cancer 30A: 1905–7, 1994

96. Hanks J. W., De Conno F., Ripamonti C., Ventafridda V., Hanna M., McQuay H. J., Mercadante S., Meynadier J., Poulain P., Roca i Casas J.: Morphine in cancer pain: modes of administration. Br Med J 312: 823–6, 1996

97. Ventafridda V., Spoldi E., Caraceni A., Tamburini M., De Conno F.: The importance of subcutaneous morphine administration for cancer pain control. Pain Clin 1: 47–55, 1986

98. Coyle N., Mauskop A., Maggard J.: Continuous subcutaneous infusions of opiates in cancer patients with pain. Oncol Nurs Forum 13: 53–7, 1986

99. Bruera E., Brenneis C., Michaud M., Bacovsky R., Chadwick S., Emeno A., MacDonald N.: Use of the subcutaneous route for the administration of narcotics in patients with cancer pain. Cancer 62: 407–11, 1988

100. Macmillan K., Bruera E., Kuehn N., Selmser P., Macmillan A.: A prospective comparison study between a butterfly needle and a teflon cannula for subcutaneous narcotic administration. J Pain Symptom Manage 9: 82–4, 1994

101. Portenoy R. K.: Continuous intravenous infusions of opioid drugs. Med Clin N Am 71: 233–41, 1987

102. Portenoy R. K., Foley K. M., Inturrisi C. E.: The nature of opioid responsiveness and its implications for neuropathic pain: new hypotheses derived from studies of opioid infusions. Pain 43: 273–86, 1990

103. Kerr I. G., Sone M., Deangelis C., Iscoe N., MacKenzie R., Schueller T.: Continuous narcotic infusion with patient-controlled analgesia for chronic cancer pain in outpatients. Ann Intern Med 108: 554–7, 1988

104. Bruera E., Macmillan K., Selmser P., Mac D. R.: Decreased local toxicity with subcutaneous diamorphine (heroin): a preliminary report. Pain 43: 91–4, 1990

105. Bruera E., Fainsinger R., Moore M., Thibault R., Spoldi E., Ventafridda V.: Local toxicity with subcutaneous methadone. Experience of two centers. Pain 45: 141–5, 1991

106. Moulin D. E., Kreeft J. H., Murray P. N., Bouquillon A. I.: Comparison of continuous subcutaneous and intravenous hydromorphone infusions for management of cancer pain. Lancet 337: 465–8, 1991

107. Storey P., Hill H. H., St. Louis R., Tarver E. E.: Subcutaneous infusions for control of cancer symptoms. J Pain Symptom Manage 5: 33–41, 1990

108. Swanson G., Smith J., Bulich R., New P., Shiffman R.: Patient-controlled analgesia for chronic cancer pain in the ambulatory setting: a report of 117 patients. J Clin Oncol 7: 1903–8, 1989

109. Hill H. F., Chapman C. R., Kornell J., Sullivan K., Saeger L., Benedetti C.: Self-administration of morphine in bone marrow transplant patients reduces drug requirement. Pain 40: 121–9, 1990

110. Hill H. F., Saeger L., Bjurstrom R., Donaldson G., Chapman C. R., Jacobson R.: Steady-state infusions of opioids in human volunteers. I. Pharmacokinetic tailoring. Pain 43: 57–69, 1991

111. Hill H. F., Coda B. A., Mackie A. M., Iverson K.: Patient-controlled analgesic infusions: alfentanil versus morphine. Pain 49: 301–10, 1992

112. Citron M., Johnston-Early A., Boyer M., Brasnow S., Hood M., Cohen M.: Patient-controlled analgesia for severe cancer pain. Arch Intern Med 146: 734–6, 1986

113. Bruera E., Brenneis C., Michaud M., MacMillan K., Hanson J., MacDonald R. N.: Patient-controlled subcutaneous hydromorphone versus continuous subcutaneous infusion for the treatment of cancer pain. J Natl Cancer Inst 80: 1152–4, 1988

114. Vanier M. C., Labrecque G., Lepage S. D., Poulin E., Provencher L., Lamontagne C.: Comparison of hydromorphone continuous subcutaneous infusion and basal rate subcutaneous infusion plus PCA in cancer pain: a pilot study. Pain 53: 27–32, 1993

115. Nordberg G.: Pharmacokinetics aspects for spinal morphine analgesia. Acta Anesthesiol Scand Suppl 28: 1984

116. Vainio A., Tigerstedt I.: Opioid treatment for radiating cancer pain: oral administration vs. epidural techniques. Acta Anaesthesiol Scand 32: 179–80, 1988

117. Max M. B., Inturrisi C. E., Kaiko R. F., Grabinski P. Y., Li C. H., Foley K. M.: Epidural and intrathecal opiates: cerebrospinal fluid and plasma profiles in patients with chronic cancer pain. Clin Pharmacol Ther 38: 631–41, 1985

118. Shetter A. G., Hadley M. N., Wilkinson E.: Administration of intraspinal morphine sul-

phate for the treatment of incurable cancer pain. Neurosurgery 18: 740–7, 1986

119. Tanelian D. L., Cousins M. J.: Failure of epidural opioid to control cancer pain in a patient previously treated with massive doses of intravenous opioid. Pain 36: 359–62, 1989

120. Hogan Q., Haddox J. D., Abram S., Weissman D., Taylor M. L., Janjan N.: Epidural opiates and local anesthetics for the management of cancer pain. Pain 46: 271–279, 1991

121. Waldman S. D., Feldstein G. S., Allen M. L.: Troubleshooting intraspinal narcotic delivery systems. Am J Nurs 87: 63–4, 1987

122. Waldman S. D., Coombs D. W.: Selection of implantable narcotic delivery systems. Anesth Analg 68: 377–84, 1989

123. Miser A. W., Narang P. K., Dothage J. A., Young R. C., Sindelar W., Miser J. S.: Transdermal fentanyl for pain control in patients with cancer. Pain 37: 15–21, 1989

124. Simmonds M. A., Richenbacher J.: Transdermal fentanyl: long-term analgesic studies. J Pain Symptom Manage 7: 536–539, 1992

125. Zech D. F., Grond S. U., Lynch J., Dauer H. G., Stollenwerk B., Lehmann K. A.: Transdermal fentanyl and initial dose-finding with patient-controlled analgesia in cancer pain. A pilot study with 20 terminally ill cancer patients. Pain 50: 293–301, 1992

126. Portenoy P. K., Southam M., Gupta S. K., Lapin J., Layman M., Inturrisi C. E., Foley K. M.: Transdermal fentanyl for cancer pain repeated dose pharmacokinetics. Anesthesiology 78: 36–43, 1993

127. Korte W., de Stoutz N., Morant R.: Day-to-day titration to initiate transdermal fentanyl in patients with cancer pain: short- and long-term experiences in a prospective study of 39 patients. J Pain Symptom Manage 11: 139–46, 1996

127a. Ahmedzai S., Brooks D.J., Group T.-f.T.: TTS-fentanyl vs oral morphine in cancer pain. Eur J Cancer 31A (Suppl 5): S182, 1995

127b. TTS Fentanyl Multicentre Study Group: Transdermal fentanyl in cancer pain. J Drug Dev 6: 93–97, 1994

127c. Donner B., Zenz M., Tryba M., Strumpf M.: Direct conversion from oral morphine to transdermal fentanyl: a multicenter study in patients with cancer pain. Pain 64: 527–534, 1996

128. Bruera E., Schoeller T., Fainsinger R. L., Kastelan C.: Custom-made suppositories of methadone for severe cancer pain. J Pain Symptom Manage 7: 372–4, 1992

129. De Conno F., Ripamonti C., Saita L., MacEachern T., Hanson J., Bruera E.: Role of rectal route in treating cancer pain: a randomized cross-over clinical trial of oral versus rectal morphine administration in opioid-naive cancer patients with pain. J Clin Oncol 13: 1004–8, 1995

130. Hanning C. D.: The rectal absorption of opioids. In: Benedetti, C., Chapman, C. R. and Giron, G. (eds): Opioid Analgesia, 14, Raven Press, New York, 1990, pp 259–69

131. Ripamonti C., Zecca E., Brunelli C., Rizio E., Saita L., Lodi F., De Conno F.: Rectal methadone in cancer patients with pain. A preliminary clinical and pharmacokinetic study. Ann Oncol 6: 841–3, 1995

132. De Conno F., Ripamonti C., Sbanotto A., Barletta L.: A clinical note on sublingual buprenorphine. J Palliat Care 9: 44–6, 1993

133. Fine P. G., Marcus M., DeBoer A. J., Van der Oord B.: An open label study of oral transmucosal fentanyl citrate (OTFC) for the treatment of breakthrough cancer pain. Pain 45: 149–55, 1991

134. Sykes N. P.: Oral naloxone in opioid associated constipation. Lancet 337: 1475, 1991

135. Culpepper-Morgan J. A., Inturrisi C. E., Portenoy R. K., Foley K. M., Houde R. W., Marsh F., Kreek M. J.: Treatment of opioid induced constipation with oral naloxone: a pilot study. Clin Pharmacol Ther 52: 90–5, 1992

136. Campora E., Merlini L., Pace M., Bruzzone M., Luzzani M., Gottlieb A., Rosso R.: The incidence of narcotic-induced emesis. J Pain Symptom Manage 6: 428–30, 1991

137. Galer B. S., Coyle N., Pasternak G. W., Portenoy R. K.: Individual variability in the response to different opioids: report of five cases. Pain 49: 87–91, 1992

138. Mac D. N., Der L., Allan S., Champion P.: Opioid hyperexcitability: the application of alternate opioid therapy. Pain 53: 353–5, 1993

139. de Stoutz N. D., Bruera E., Suarez-Aimazor M.: Opiate rotation (OR) for toxicity reduction in terminal cancer patients. 7th World Congress on Pain: Congress Abstracts,

I.A.S.P. Publications, Seattle, 1993, pp abstract 894

140. Cherny N. J., Chang V., Frager G., Ingham J. M., Tiseo P., Popp B., Portenoy R. K., Foley K. M.: Opioid pharmacotherapy in the management of cancer pain. A survey of strategies used by pain physicians for the selection of analgesic drugs and routes of administration. Cancer 76: 1288–93, 1995

141. Ettinger D. S., Vitale P. J., Trump D. L.: Important clinical pharmacological considerations in the use of methadone in cancer patients. Cancer Treat Rep 63: 457–9, 1979

142. Plummer J. L., Gourlay G. K., Cherry D. A., Cousins M. J.: Estimation of methadone clearance: application in the management of cancer pain. Pain 33: 313–22, 1988

143. Bruera E., Watanabe S., Faisinger R. L., Spachynski K., Suarez-Almazor M., Inturrisi C.: Custom-made capsules and suppositories of methadone for patients on high-dose opioids for cancer pain. Pain 62: 141–6, 1995

144. Jadad A. R., Carroll D., Glynn C. J., Moore R. A., McQuay H. J.: Morphine responsiveness of chronic pain: double blind randomised crossover study with patient controlled analgesia. Lancet 339: 1367–71, 1992

145. Banning A., Sjogren P., Henriksen H.: Treatment outcome in a multidisciplinary cancer pain. Pain 47: 129–34, 1991

146. Du Pen S., Kharasch E. D., Williams A., Peterson D. G., Sloan D. C., Hasche K. H., Krembs A. W.: Chronic epidural bupivacaine-opioid infusion in intractable cancer pain. Pain 49: 293–300, 1992

147. Sjoberg M., Appelgren L., Einarsson S., Hultman E., Linder L. E., Nitescu P., Curelaru I.: Long-term intrathecal morphine and bupivacaine in "refractory" cancer pain. Results from the first series of 52 patients. Acta Anaesthesiol Scand 35: 30–43, 1991

148. Max M. B.: Antidepressants as analgesics. In: Fields, H. L. and Liebeskind, J. C. (eds): Pharmacological approaches in the treatment of chronic pain: new concepts and critical issues. Progress in pain research and management vol.1, IASP Press, Seattle, 1994, pp 229–46

149. Galer B. S.: Neuropathic pain of peripheral origin: advances in pharmacologic treatment. Neurology 45(Suppl 9): S17–S25, 1995

150. Watson C. P., Chipman M., Reed K., Evans R. J., Birkett N.: Amitriptyline versus maprotiline in postherpetic neuralgia: a randomized, double-blind, crossover trial. Pain 48: 29–36, 1992

151. McQuay H., Carroll D., Jadad A. R., Wiffen P., Moore A.: Anticonvulsant drugs for management of pain: a systematic review. Br Med J 311: 1047–52, 1995

152. Tanelian D. L., Cousins M. J.: Combined neurogenic and nociceptive pain in a patient with Pancoast tumor managed by epidural hydromorphone and oral carbamazepine. Pain 36: 85–8, 1989

153. Fromm G. H., Terrence C. F., Chattha A. S.: Baclofen in the treatment of trigeminal neuralgia: double-blind study and long-term follow-up. Ann Neurol 15: 240–4, 1984

154. Twycross R.: Corticosteroids in advanced cancer [editorial; comment]. Br Med J 305: 969–70, 1992

155. Ettinger A. B., Portenoy R. K.: The use of corticosteroids in the treatment of symptoms associated with cancer. J Pain Symptom Manage 3: 99–103, 1988

156. Greenberg H. S., Kim J., Posner J. B.: Epidural spinal cord compression from metastatic tumor: results with a new treatment protocol. Ann Neurol 8: 361–6, 1980

157. Vecht C. J., Haaxma–Reiche H., van Putten W. L. J., de Visser M., Vries E. P., Twijnstra A.: Initial bolus of conventional versus high-dose dexamethasone in metastatic spinal cord compression. Neurology 39: 1255–7, 1989

158. Marchettini P., Lacerenza M., Marangoni C., et al.: Lidocaine test in neuralgia. Pain 48: 377–82, 1992

159. Dejgard A., Petersen P., Kastrup J.: Mexiletine for treatment of chronic painful diabetic neuropathy. Lancet 1: 9–11, 1988

160. Chabal C., Jacobson L., Mariano A., Chaney E., Britell C. W.: The use of oral mexiletine for the treatment of pain after peripheral nerve injury. Anesthesiology 76: 513–17, 1992

161. Brose W. G., Cousins M. J.: Subcutaneous lidocaine for treatment of neuropathic cancer pain. Pain 45: 145–8, 1991

162. Ventafridda V., Ripamonti C., Caraceni A., Spoldi E., Messina L., De Conno F.: The management of inoperable gastrointestinal obstruction in terminal cancer patients. Tumori 76: 389–93, 1990

58

163. Mercadante S., Spoldi E., Caraceni A., Maddaloni S., Simonetti M. T.: Octreotide in relieving gastrointestinal symptoms due to bowel obstruction. Palliat Med 7: 295–9, 1993

164. Harvey A. H., Lipton A.: The role of bisphosphonates in the treatment of bone metastases – the US experience. Support Care Cancer 4: 213–17, 1996

165. Thurlimann B., Morant R., Jungi W. F., Radziwill A.: Pamidronate for pain control in patients with malignant osteolytic bone disease: a prospective dose effect study. Support Care Cancer 1: 61–5, 1994

166. Berenson J. R., Lichtenstein A., Porter L., et al.: Efficacy of pamidronate in reducing skeletal events in patients with advanced multiple myeloma. N Engl J Med 334: 488–93, 1996

167. Bataille R.: Management of myeloma with bisphosphonates. N Engl J Med 334: 530–1, 1996

168. Ventafridda V., Caraceni A.: Cancer Pain. In: Prithvi Raj, P. (ed.): Current review of pain, Current Medicine, Philadelphia, 1994, pp 156–78

169. Lipton S.: Neurodestructive procedures in the management of cancer pain. J Pain Symptom Manage 2: 219–28, 1987

170. Ventafridda V., Tamburini M., De Conno F.: Comprehensive treatment in cancer pain. In: Fields, H. L. et al. (eds): Advances in Pain Research and Therapy, vol. 9, Raven Press, New York, 1985, pp 617–28

171. Ischia S., Ischia A., Polati E., Finco G.: Three posterior percutaneous celiac plexus block techniques. A prospective, randomized study in 61 patients with pancreatic cancer pain. Anesthesiology 76: 534–40, 1992

172. Mercadante S.: Celiac plexus block versus analgesics in pancreatic cancer pain. Pain 52: 187–92, 1993

173. Loeser J. D.: Neurosurgical approaches in palliative care. In: Doyle, D., Hanks, J. W. and MacDonald, N. (eds): Oxford Textbook of Palliative Medicine, Oxford University Press, Oxford, 1993, pp 221–29

174. Swarm R. A., Cousins M. J.: Anesthetic techniques for pain control. In: Doyle, D., Hanks, G. W. and MacDonald, N. (eds): Oxford Textbook of Palliative Medicine, Oxford University Press, Oxford, 1993, pp 204–21

175. Eisenberg E., Carr D. B., Chalmers T. C.: Neurolytic celiac plexus for treatment of cancer pain. Anesth Analg 80: 290–5, 1995

175a. Kawamata M., Ishtani K., Ishikawa K., Sasaki H., Ota K., Omote K.: Comparison between celiac plexus block and morphine treatment on quality of life in patients with pancreatic cancer pain. Pain 64: 597–602, 1996

175b. Ventafridda G., Caraceni A., Sbanotto A.M., Barletta L., De C.F.: Pain treatment in cancer of the pancreas. Eur J Surg Oncol 16:1–6, 1990

175c. De Conno F., Caraceni A., Aldrighetti L., Magnani G., Ferla G., Comi G.: Paraplegia following coeliac plexus block. Pain 55: 383–385, 1993

175d. Ventafridda V., Fochi C., Sganzerla E. et al.: Neurolitic blocks in perineal pain. In: Bonica J.J., Ventafridda V. (eds): Advances in Pain Research and Therapy Vol.2., Raven Press: New York, 1979, PP 597–605

176. Ischia S., Ischia A., Luzzani A., Toscano D., Steele A.: Results up to death in the treatment of persistent cervico-thoracic (Pancoast) and thoracic malignant pain by unilateral percutaneous cervical cordotomy. Pain 21: 339–55, 1985

177. Sanders M., Zuurmond W.: Safety of unilateral and bilateral percutaneous cervical cordotomy in 80 terminally ill cancer patients. J Clin Oncol 13: 1509 –12, 1995

RECOMMENDED LITERATURE

Cancer pain epidemiology and characteristics

1. Greenwald H. P., Bonica J. J., Bergner M.: The prevalence of pain in four cancers. Cancer 60: 2563–9, 1987
2. Portenoy R. K., Kornblith A. B., Wong G., Vlamis V., McCarthy Lepore J., Loseth D. B., Hakes T., Foley K. M., Hoskins W. J.: Pain in ovarian cancer patients. Prevalence, characteristics, and associated symptoms. Cancer 74: 907–15, 1994
3. Portenoy R. K., Miransky J., Thaler H. T., Hornung J., Bianchi C., Cibas-Kong I., Feldhamer E., Lewis F., Matamoros I., Sugar M. Z., Olivieri A. P., Kemeny N. E., Foley K. M.: Pain in ambulatory patients with lung and colon cancer. Prevalence, characteristics, and effect. Cancer 70: 1616–24, 1992
4. Greenwald H. P.: Interethnic differences in pain perception. Pain 44: 157–63, 1991
5. Cleeland C. S., Gonin R., Hatfield A. K., Edmonson J. H., Blum R. H., Stewart J. A., Pandya K. J.: Pain and its treatment in outpatients with metastatic cancer. N Engl J Med 330: 592–6, 1994
6. Grond S., Zech D., Diefenbach C., Radbruch L., Lehman K. A.: Assessment of cancer pain: a prospective evaluation in 2266 cancer patients referred to a pain service. Pain 64: 107–14, 1996

Assessment and measurement

7. Cleeland C. S., Ladinsky J. L., Serlin R. C., Nugyen C. T.: Multidimensional measurement of cancer pain: comparisons of US and Vietnamese patients. J Pain Symptom Manage 3: 23–7, 1988
8. Bookbinder M., Kiss M., Coyle N., Gianella A., Thaler H. T.: Improving pain management practice. In: McGuire, D. B., Henke Yarbro, C. and Rolling Ferrell, B. (eds): Cancer Pain Management, Jones and Bartlett, Boston, 1995, pp 321–61

9. Foley K. M.: Pain assessment and cancer pain syndromes. In: Doyle, D., Hanks, G. W. and MacDonald, N. (eds): Oxford Textbook of Palliative Medicine, Oxford University Press, Oxford, 1993, pp 148–65

Anatomy and physiology of the nociceptive system

10. Willis W. D. The Pain System: The Neural Basis of Nociceptive Transmission in the Mammalian Nervous System. Basel: Karger, 1985

Neuropathic pain pathophysiology

11. Willis W. Hyperalgesia and allodynia. New York: Raven Press, 1992

Cancer pain syndromes in general

12. Cherny N. I., Portenoy R. K.: Cancer Pain: principles of assessment and syndromes. In: Wall, P. D. and Melzack, R. (eds): Textbook of Pain, Churchill Livingstone, Edinburgh, 1994, pp 787–823
13. Elliot K. J.: Taxonomy and mechanisms of neuropathic pain. Semin Neurol 14: 195–205, 1994
14. Elliott S. C., Miser A. W., Dose A. M., Betcher D. L., O'Fallon J. R., Ducos R. S., Shah N. R., Goh T. S., Monzon C. M., Tschetter L.: Epidemiologic features of pain in pediatric cancer patients: a co-operative community-based study. North Central Cancer Treatment Group and Mayo Clinic. Clin J Pain 7: 263–8, 1991
15. Caraceni A.: Clinicopathological correlates of common cancer pain syndromes. Hematol Oncol Clin N Am 10: 57–78, 1996

Spinal cord compression

16. Posner I. B.: Back pain and epidural spinal cord compression. Med Clin N Am 71: 185–206, 1987
17. Byrne T. N., Waxman S. G.: Spinal cord compression: diagnosis and principles of treatment. Philadelphia: F.A. Davis, 1990
18. Byrne T. N.: Spinal Metastases. In: Wiley, R. G. (ed.): Neurological complications of cancer, Marcel Dekker, New York, 1995, pp 23–44

Brachial plexopathy

19. Foley K.: Brachial plexopathy in patients with breast cancer. In: Harris, J. R., Hellman, S., Henderson, I. C. and Kinne, D. (eds): Breast Diseases., Lippincott, Philadelphia, 1991, pp 722–9

Polyneuropathy, leptomeningeal metastases, plexopathy

20. Henson R. A., Urich H.: Cancer and the Nervous System. Blackwell Scientific Publications, Boston, 1982, pp 100–19, 368–405
21. Posner J. B.: Neurologic complications of cancer. Philadelphia: F.A. Davis, 1995
22. Wiley R. G. (ed.): Neurological complications of cancer. New York: Marcel Dekker, 1995

Opioid pharmacology and pharmacotherapy

23. Foley K. M.: Controversies in cancer pain: medical perspective. Cancer 63: 2257–65, 1989
24. Foley K. M., Inturrisi C. E.: Opioid analgesics in the management of clinical pain. New York: Raven Press, 1986
25. Cherny N. I., Portenoy R. K.: Practical issues in the management of cancer pain. In: Wall, P. D. and Melzack, R. (eds): Textbook of Pain, Edinburgh: Churchill Livingstone, 1994, pp 1437–67
26. Woodruff R.: Palliative Treatment. Victoria, Australia: Asperula Pty. Ltd., 1993

Analgesics for neuropathic pain

27a. Fields H. L., Liebeskind J. C.: Pharmacological approaches to the treatment of chronic pain: new concepts and critical issues. Seattle: IASP Press, 1994
27b. Portenoy R.K., Kanner R.H.: Pain Management: Theory and Practice. Philadelphia: F.A. Davis, 1996

Invasive techniques

28. Patt R.: Cancer Pain. Philadelphia: J.B. Lippincott, 1993
29. Ventafridda V., Caraceni A.: Cancer Pain. In: Prithvi Raj, P. (ed.): Current review of pain, Current Medicine, Philadelphia, 1994, pp 156–78